Fast Facts

Fast Facts:
Epilepsy

Third edition

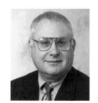

Martin J Brodie MB ChB MRCP MD FRCP
Director, Epilepsy Unit
Division of Cardiovascular and Medical Sciences
Western Infirmary
Glasgow, UK

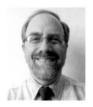

Steven C Schachter MS MD FAAN
Director of Research, Department of Neurology
Beth Israel Deaconess Medical Center
Professor of Neurology, Harvard Medical School
Boston, Massachusetts, USA

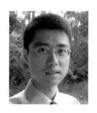

Patrick Kwan MD PhD
Associate Consultant and Honorary Associate Professor
Division of Neurology, Department of Medicine & Therapeutics
The Chinese University of Hong Kong
Prince of Wales Hospital
Shatin, Hong Kong

Declaration of Independence

This book is as balanced and as practical as we can make it.
Ideas for improvement are always welcome:
feedback@fastfacts.com

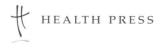

HEALTH PRESS

Fast Facts – Epilepsy
First published 1999
Second edition 2001
Third edition September 2005

Text © 2005 Martin J Brodie, Steven C Schachter, Patrick Kwan
© 2005 in this edition Health Press Limited
Health Press Limited, Elizabeth House, Queen Street, Abingdon,
Oxford OX14 3LN, UK
Tel: +44 (0)1235 523233
Fax: +44 (0)1235 523238

Book orders can be placed by telephone or via the website.
For regional distributors or to order via the website, please go to:
www.fastfacts.com
For telephone orders, please call 01752 202301 (UK), +44 1752 202301 (Europe),
800 247 6553 (USA, toll free) or 419 281 1802 (Canada).

Fast Facts is a trademark of Health Press Limited.

The authors wish to thank NC Sin, MD, Department of Paediatrics, Prince of Wales
Hospital, Hong Kong, for supplying Figure 3.4 (which is also reproduced on the
cover) and Howard L. Weiner, MD, Division of Pediatric Neurosurgery, New York
University Medical Center, New York, USA, for supplying Figures 6.1, 6.2 and 6.3.

The publisher and the authors have made every effort to ensure the accuracy of this
book, but cannot accept responsibility for any errors or omissions.

For all drugs, please consult the product labeling approved in your country for
prescribing information.

Registered names, trademarks, etc. used in this book, even when not marked as such,
are not to be considered unprotected by law.

A CIP catalogue record for this title is available from the British Library.

ISBN 1-903734-30-4

Brodie, MJ (Martin)
Fast Facts – Epilepsy/
Martin J Brodie, Steven C Schachter, Patrick Kwan

Medical illustrations by Annamaria Dutto, Withernsea, UK.
Typesetting and page layout by Zed, Oxford, UK.
Printed by Fine Print (Services) Ltd, Oxford, UK.

Printed with vegetable inks on fully biodegradable and
recyclable paper manufactured from sustainable forests.

444   001
Low emissions
during production

Low   Sustainable
chlorine   forests

Abbreviations

ACTH: adrenocorticotropic hormone

AED: antiepileptic drug

CBZ: carbamazepine

CLB: clobazam

CNS: central nervous system

CT: computed tomography

CYP: cytochrome P450

CZP: clonazepam

DEXA: dual-energy X-ray absorptiometry

DSM IV: *Diagnostic and Statistical Manual of Mental Disorders*, fourth edition

EEG: electroencephalogram

ESM: ethosuximide

FBM: felbamate

GABA: gamma-aminobutyric acid

GBP: gabapentin

GTCS: generalized tonic–clonic seizures

HS: hippocampal sclerosis

JME: juvenile myoclonic epilepsy

LEV: levetiracetam

LTG: lamotrigine

MRI: magnetic resonance imaging

MTLE: mesial temporal lobe epilepsy

NTZ: nitrazepam

OXC: oxcarbazepine

PB: phenobarbital

PET: positron emission tomography

PGB: pregabalin

PHT: phenytoin

PRM: primidone

SE: status epilepticus

SSRI: selective serotonin reuptake inhibitor

SUDEP: sudden unexpected death in epilepsy

TCA: tricyclic antidepressant

TGB: tiagabine

TPM: topiramate

VGB: vigabatrin

VNS: vagus nerve stimulation

VPA: sodium valproate

ZNS: zonisamide

Glossary

Cryptogenic epilepsy: epilepsy presumed to have an underlying anatomic cause that remains unidentified

Cytochrome P450: a family of isoenzymes responsible for the hepatic oxidation of a range of lipid-soluble drugs

Enzyme inducer: a drug that increases synthesis of drug-metabolizing enzymes

Epilepsy: a chronic disorder of the brain characterized by an enduring disposition toward recurrent unprovoked seizures

Epilepsy syndrome: a constellation of characteristic seizures, abnormalities on EEG and/or brain imaging, response to therapy, prognosis, and associated clinical history and/or examination findings

Epileptogenesis: a sequence of events that converts a normal neuronal network into a hyperexcitable one

Generalized seizures: seizures that initially involve both hemispheres, usually with impairment of consciousness at the outset

Half-life: time taken for the plasma concentration of a drug to drop by 50%

Hypsarrhythmia: EEG pattern associated with infantile spasms, characterized by diffuse high-voltage spike-and-slow-wave complexes, superimposed on a disorganized, slow background

Idiopathic epilepsy: epilepsy that has a probable genetic basis

Incidence: the number of people developing epilepsy within a given time

Interictal: between epileptic seizures

Lennox–Gastaut syndrome: an encephalopathic syndrome of early childhood involving multiple seizure types, major abnormalities on EEG and usually mental retardation

Localization-related epilepsy: epilepsy with partial-onset seizures (also called focal epilepsy)

Non-epileptic seizure event: a non-epileptic event that mimics a seizure without any identifiable physiological abnormality (also called a pseudoseizure or psychogenic seizure)

Partial seizure: a sudden, excessive, rapid and localized electrical discharge by gray matter from a particular part of the brain with ('complex partial') or without ('simple partial') impairment of consciousness

Pharmacogenomics: pharmacological targets identified from genetic mutations underlying epilepsy syndromes

Prevalence: the number of people with a diagnosis of epilepsy at any time

Seizure: transient symptoms and/or signs due to abnormal excessive or synchronous activity of a population of cortical neurons

Status epilepticus: continued or repeated seizure activity

Steady state: the concentration of drug achieved when the rate of administration equals the rate of elimination, after around five elimination half-lives

Stevens–Johnson syndrome: severe idiosyncratic reaction characterized by skin eruption and mucosal and endothelial damage

Symptomatic epilepsy: epilepsy with an identified underlying cause

West syndrome: a rare condition characterized by the triad of infantile spasms, a typical hypsarrhythmic EEG pattern and arrest of psychomotor development

Introduction

Epilepsy – derived from the Greek word *epilambanein*, meaning 'to seize' or 'to attack' – was first recorded in the West in a Babylonian treatise discovered in southern Turkey. The disorder was later recognized in classical Chinese medical texts written from 770 to 221 BC. Around 400 BC, Hippocrates described epilepsy as 'the sacred disease', but most cultures placed a demoniac interpretation on its unique constellation of symptoms and signs. It was only in 1875 that the English neurologist John Hughlings Jackson recognized a seizure as being due to disordered brain electricity.

Epilepsy is the most common serious neurological disorder in the world. Although this distressing condition remits in some people, many will have epilepsy throughout their lives. It affects all ages and crosses all geographic boundaries.

There have been a number of scientific and sociological revolutions surrounding this common yet previously much-neglected disorder. These have been fueled by:
- advances in molecular biology
- better understanding of the pathophysiology of seizure propagation and generation
- appreciation of a widening range of seizure types and epilepsy syndromes
- development of more precise and accurate brain imaging techniques
- new antiepileptic drugs (AEDs) with different mechanisms of action
- better use of epilepsy surgery in patients with medically intractable seizures.

One of the more exciting recent developments is the slow unraveling of the genetics that underpin the mechanisms of neuronal excitation and inhibition.

We have extensively revised this third edition of *Fast Facts – Epilepsy*, including updated illustrations, to incorporate the rapid advances being made in our understanding of this debilitating disorder. With regards to pharmacological management, we have included a section on the principles of AED selection along with the latest information on the

AEDs now available. The chapter on non-pharmacological management includes new information pertaining to the ketogenic diet and alternative medicine. We have also added information specific to women with epilepsy, and have included a new chapter that covers the psychiatric morbidities and social aspects of the disorder.

Although this handbook has inevitably 'grown' as a result of these revisions, we hope it will remain a succinct and practical aid for clinicians to diagnose and successfully treat people with a wide range of seizure disorders.

Incidence and prevalence

Around 50 million people in the world have epilepsy. It is the commonest serious neurological condition, with an annual incidence in developed countries of 50–70 cases per 100 000 of the population (Figure 1.1).

In developing countries, the figure is higher due to more primitive obstetric services and consequently the greater likelihood of cerebral infection and head trauma.

The point prevalence of epilepsy is around 1% in both developing and developed countries.

Incidence varies greatly with age, with high rates in early childhood, low levels in early adult life and a second peak in people aged over 65 years old (Figure 1.2).

In recent years, there has been a fall in the number of affected children accompanied by a sharp rise in epilepsy in the elderly. Indeed, old age has become the most common time in life to develop the condition.

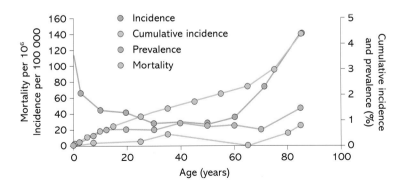

Figure 1.1 Incidence, prevalence, cumulative incidence and mortality for epilepsy in Rochester, Minnesota, 1935–1984. Reproduced with permission from Hauser WA et al. *Mayo Clin Proc* 1996;71:576–86.

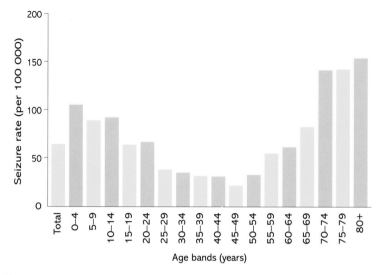

Figure 1.2 Incidence of epilepsy in relation to age. Reproduced with permission from Oxford University Press from Tallis et al. 1991.

Prognosis

The majority of patients with epilepsy have a good prognosis. The prognosis is strongly influenced by the underlying cause. In many people, particularly children, the condition will remit, although a substantial proportion will have epilepsy all their lives. Overall, 60–70% of patients become seizure free after treatment with antiepileptic drugs (AEDs), and some patients can remain in remission after subsequent drug withdrawal. The other 30–40% continue to have seizures with varying degrees of frequency and severity. Factors that indicate a poor prognosis include:

• symptomatic cause
• high seizure frequency before AED treatment
• generalized tonic–clonic seizures
• generalized epileptiform activity on the electroencephalogram
• family history of epilepsy
• comorbid psychiatric history.

Recent data suggest that poor long-term outcome can be predicted if seizures are not controlled after two consecutive AED treatment schedules owing to lack of efficacy.

Mortality

The standardized mortality ratio (the number of observed deaths per number of expected deaths) for patients with epilepsy is 2–3 times above that of the general population. In many cases, the cause of death is related to the underlying etiology, but sudden unexpected death in epilepsy (SUDEP) is now believed to account for up to 17% of all epilepsy-related deaths. SUDEP has been defined as 'sudden, unexpected, witnessed or unwitnessed, non-traumatic and non-drowning death in patients with epilepsy, with or without evidence of a seizure, and excluding documented status epilepticus, in which postmortem examination does not reveal toxicological or anatomic cause of death'. The reported incidence of SUDEP varies from 0.35 to 10 per 1000 patients per year. It is higher if the seizure disorder remains uncontrolled, suggesting that the majority of SUDEP is related to seizure activity. Other associated causes of death include drowning, burns, aspiration, pneumonia, status epilepticus and suicide.

Key points – epidemiology and prognosis

- Epilepsy is the commonest serious neurological disorder.
- The incidence of epilepsy is highest in the elderly.
- Epilepsy can be controlled by antiepileptic drugs in the majority of patients.
- People with epilepsy have a mortality 2–3 times greater than the expected number of deaths in the general population.

Key references

Annegers JF, Rocca WA, Hauser WA. Causes of epilepsy: contributions of the Rochester epidemiology project. *Mayo Clin Proc* 1996;71:570–5.

Bell GS, Sander JW. The epidemiology of epilepsy: the size of the problem. *Seizure* 2001;10:306–16.

Jallon P. Mortality in patients with epilepsy. *Curr Opin Neurol* 2004;17:141–6.

Kotsopoulos IA, van Merode T, Kessels FG et al. Systematic review and meta-analysis of incidence studies of epilepsy and unprovoked seizures. *Epilepsia* 2002;43:1402–9.

Kwan P, Brodie MJ. Early identification of refractory epilepsy. *N Engl J Med* 2000;342:314–19.

Kwan P, Sander JW. The natural history of epilepsy: an epidemiological view. *J Neurol Neurosurg Psychiatry* 2004;75: 1376–81.

Perucca E. Pharmacoresistance in epilepsy: how should it be defined? *CNS Drugs* 1998;10:171–9.

Tallis R, Hall G, Craig I, Dean A. How common are epileptic seizures in old age? *Age Ageing* 1991;20: 442–8.

Tomson T, Beghi E, Sundqvist A, Johannessen SI. Medical risks in epilepsy: a review with focus on physical injuries, mortality, traffic accidents and their prevention. *Epilepsy Res* 2004;60:1–16.

Seizure types

A seizure is a symptom and represents the clinical manifestation of an abnormal and excessive synchronized discharge of a set of cortical neurons in the brain. Establishing the type(s) of seizure experienced by the patient has important implications for:

- selection of antiepileptic drugs (AEDs)
- likelihood of an underlying cerebral lesion
- prognosis
- possible genetic transmission.

Depending on the pattern of neuronal involvement, the clinical features of a seizure consist of a wide range of sudden and transitory abnormal phenomena, which may include alterations of consciousness, or motor, sensory, autonomic or psychic events. The present electroclinical classification of seizures established by the International League Against Epilepsy (ILAE) is the most widely adopted scheme. This classification system, viewed by the ILAE as a work in progress, divides seizures into two major groups: partial and generalized (Table 2.1).

Partial seizures originate in a focal region of the cortex (Figure 2.1) and can be subdivided into those that do not impair consciousness (simple partial) and those that do (complex partial). Both types of partial seizure can spread rapidly to other cortical areas through neuronal networks, resulting in secondary generalized tonic–clonic seizures (Figure 2.2).

Simple partial seizures. The symptoms and signs of simple partial seizures depend on the site of origin of the abnormal electrical discharge. For example, those arising from the motor cortex cause rhythmic movements of the contralateral face, arm or leg (formerly called Jacksonian seizures). Seizures arising from sensory regions or areas responsible for emotions and memory may produce olfactory, visual or auditory hallucinations, feelings of déjà vu or jamais vu, or fear, panic or euphoria.

TABLE 2.1

International classification of epileptic seizures*

Partial seizures (beginning locally)	Generalized seizures (convulsive or non-convulsive)
Simple partial (without impaired consciousness)	Absence
–with motor symptoms	– typical
– with somatosensory or special sensory symptoms	– atypical
– with autonomic symptoms	Myoclonic
– with psychic symptoms	Clonic
Complex partial (with impaired consciousness)	Tonic
	Tonic–clonic
– simple partial onset followed by impaired consciousness	Atonic
	Unclassified
– impaired consciousness at onset	
Partial, evolving into secondary generalized seizures	

*Adapted from Commission on Classification and Terminology of the International League Against Epilepsy, 1981.

Complex partial seizures, previously called temporal lobe or psychomotor seizures, are the most common seizure type in adults and the most difficult to control with treatment. There may be a warning, called an aura (simple partial seizure), immediately preceding loss or reduction of awareness. Complex partial seizures typically last less than 3 minutes. During that time, patients may appear awake, but lose contact with their environment and do not respond normally to instructions or questions. Patients usually stare and either remain motionless or engage in repetitive semi-purposeful behavior called automatisms, including facial grimacing, gesturing, chewing, lip smacking, snapping fingers, repeating words or phrases, walking, running or even undressing. Patients cannot remember behaving in this

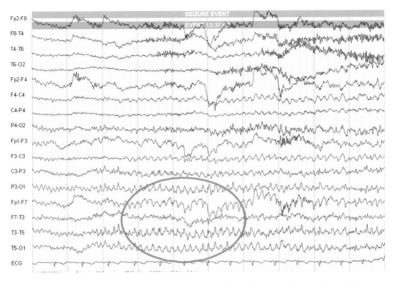

Figure 2.1 EEG showing a focal seizure over the left temporal area (circled).

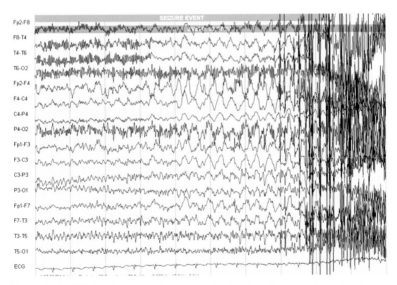

Figure 2.2 EEG showing secondary generalization from the partial-onset seizure in Figure 2.1.

manner. If restrained, they may become hostile or aggressive. After a seizure, patients are often sleepy and confused, and complain of a headache. This post-ictal state can vary from minutes to hours.

Generalized seizures are characterized by widespread involvement of bilateral cortical regions at the outset and are usually accompanied by impairment of consciousness. The familiar tonic–clonic seizure (previously called 'grand mal') is often preceded by a cry. The patient suddenly falls to the ground and exhibits typical convulsive movements, sometimes with tongue or mouth biting and urinary incontinence. Other subtypes of generalized seizures include absence, myoclonic, clonic, tonic and atonic seizures (see Table 2.1).

Absence seizures (previously called 'petit mal') mainly affect children.

Typical absence seizures usually last 5–10 seconds and commonly occur in clusters. They manifest as sudden onset of staring and impaired consciousness with or without eye blinking and lip smacking. The electroencephalogram (EEG) typically shows a 3-Hz spike-and-wave pattern (Figure 2.3). There is a strong genetic component for the seizures as well as for the EEG abnormality. While absences will remit during adolescence in around 40% of patients, related tonic–clonic seizures may continue into adulthood.

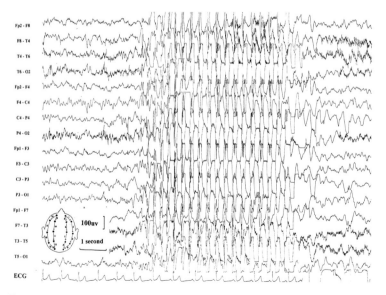

Figure 2.3 EEG showing a 3-Hz spike-and-wave pattern of a typical absence seizure, with characteristic abrupt onset and cessation.

Atypical absence seizures usually begin before 5 years of age in conjunction with other generalized seizure types and mental retardation. They last longer than typical absence seizures and are often associated with changes in muscle tone.

Myoclonic seizures consist of sudden, brief muscle contractions, either singly or in clusters, that can affect any muscle group.

Clonic seizures are characterized by rhythmic or semi-rhythmic muscle contractions, typically involving the upper extremities, neck and face.

Tonic seizures cause sudden stiffening of extensor muscles, often associated with impaired consciousness and falling to the ground.

Atonic seizures (drop attacks) produce sudden loss of muscle tone with instantaneous collapse, often resulting in facial or other injuries.

Epilepsy syndromes

In addition to the classification of seizures, there is a separate system for epilepsies and epileptic syndromes (Table 2.2). These are defined by groups of characteristic clinical features related to age of onset of seizures, family history of epilepsy, seizure type(s) and associated neurological symptoms and signs, aided by appropriate investigations, including electroencephalography and brain imaging such as computed tomography and magnetic resonance imaging (MRI) (see Chapter 3, Diagnosis).

Diagnosing an epileptic syndrome helps the clinician to define the likely prognosis, provide reasonable genetic counseling and choose the most appropriate AEDs.

Epileptic syndromes are divided into:
- localization-related or focal epilepsies (those with partial-onset seizures)
- generalized epilepsies (those with generalized seizures).

Based on the knowledge of etiology, the syndromes are then further subdivided into:
- idiopathic – presumed to be genetic in origin
- symptomatic (secondary) – of known cause
- cryptogenic – presumed to be symptomatic but with an unidentified underlying abnormality.

17

TABLE 2.2

International classification of epilepsies and epileptic syndromes*

Localization-related (focal, local or partial)

Idiopathic epilepsy with age-related onset

- benign childhood epilepsy with centrotemporal spikes
  (benign rolandic epilepsy)

- childhood epilepsy with occipital paroxysms

- primary reading epilepsy

Symptomatic epilepsy

Cryptogenic epilepsy

Generalized

Idiopathic epilepsy with age-related onset (listed in order of age
at onset)

- benign neonatal familial convulsions

- benign neonatal non-familial convulsions

- benign myoclonic epilepsy in infancy

- childhood absence epilepsy

- juvenile myoclonic epilepsy

- epilepsy with generalized tonic–clonic seizures on awakening

- other idiopathic epilepsies

Cryptogenic or symptomatic epilepsy (listed in order of age at onset)

- West syndrome (infantile spasms)

- Lennox–Gastaut syndrome (childhood epileptic encephalopathy)

- epilepsy with myoclonic–astatic seizures

- epilepsy with myoclonic absence seizures

Symptomatic epilepsy

- Non-specific syndromes (early myoclonic encephalopathy, early
  infantile epileptic encephalopathy)

- Specific syndromes (epileptic seizures as a complication of a disease,
  such as phenylketonuria, juvenile Gaucher's disease or Lundborg's
  progressive myoclonic epilepsy)

TABLE 2.2 (CONTINUED)

Epilepsies undetermined whether focal or generalized

With both generalized and focal features

- neonatal seizures

- severe myoclonic epilepsy in infancy

- epilepsy with continuous spike waves during slow-wave sleep

- acquired epileptic aphasia (Landau–Kleffner syndrome)

Without unequivocal generalized or focal features[†]

Special syndromes

Situation-related seizures

- febrile convulsions

- seizures related to other identifiable situations, such as stress, hormonal changes, drugs, alcohol withdrawal or sleep deprivation

Isolated, apparently unprovoked epileptic events

Epilepsies characterized by specific modes of seizure precipitation

Chronic progressive epilepsia partialis continua of childhood

*Adapted from Commission on Classification and Terminology of the International League Against Epilepsy, 1989.
[†]Includes cases in which the clinical and electroencephalographic findings do not permit classification of the epilepsy as clearly generalized or localization-related, such as cases of tonic–clonic seizures during sleep.

The accuracy of classification depends on the extent of investigation. With advances in technology, in particular brain imaging, many subtle lesions can now be identified, making it possible to classify more of the epilepsies as symptomatic rather than cryptogenic. Like the classification of seizures, fueled by recent developments in diagnostic imaging and molecular genetics, the classification of epilepsy syndromes is also under revision.

There are several epileptic syndromes that may be encountered by the family physician: benign rolandic epilepsy, juvenile myoclonic epilepsy, febrile convulsions, infantile spasms, Lennox–Gastaut syndrome and mesial temporal lobe epilepsy. An increasing number of single gene mutations are being recognized as unusual causes of epilepsy syndromes.

Benign rolandic epilepsy, also called benign childhood epilepsy with centrotemporal spikes, is an idiopathic focal epilepsy syndrome, with onset from age 3 to 13 years. Nocturnal seizures predominate, and patients display a characteristic EEG pattern. Affected patients usually have normal cognitive function and neurological examination findings. Seizures have a simple partial onset with occasional secondary generalization. Nocturnal seizures involve excessive salivation, gurgling or choking sounds, and clonic contractions of the mouth. Daytime seizures usually consist of tonic and/or clonic movements of one side of the body (particularly the face) and speech arrest, but the child remains conscious.

The EEG shows high-amplitude midtemporal-central spikes and sharp waves, particularly during light sleep (Figure 2.4). The prognosis for children with benign rolandic epilepsy is excellent. The seizures are generally very easy to control with AEDs. The most commonly employed AEDs tend to be carbamazepine (CBZ), valproate (VPA) and benzodiazepines given at bedtime. However, many children with mild or infrequent seizures do not require prophylactic AED treatment. Nearly all patients outgrow the disorder by their teenage years.

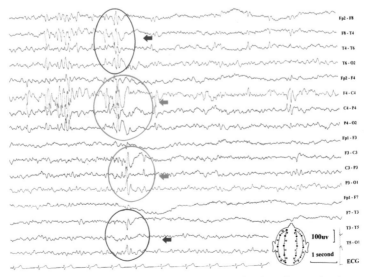

Figure 2.4 Interictal EEG of a patient with benign rolandic epilepsy showing midtemporal (blue arrows) and central (red arrows) spikes and sharp waves.

Juvenile myoclonic epilepsy (JME) is an under-recognized syndrome characterized by myoclonic jerks, tonic–clonic seizures or clonic–tonic–clonic seizures, and, occasionally, absence seizures. Myoclonic seizures occur within the first few hours after arising from sleep (as do the generalized seizures), are mild and bilaterally symmetrical, and usually involve the upper extremities without impairing consciousness. The patient may spill or drop things during a myoclonic jerk. Less commonly, myoclonic seizures affecting the legs can cause falls.

JME is an inherited condition in otherwise neurologically normal children. It usually begins during the teenage years. The EEG shows a characteristic spike-and-wave pattern of 3.5–6 Hz, and multiple spike-and-wave complexes that may be precipitated by photic stimulation and sleep deprivation (Figure 2.5).

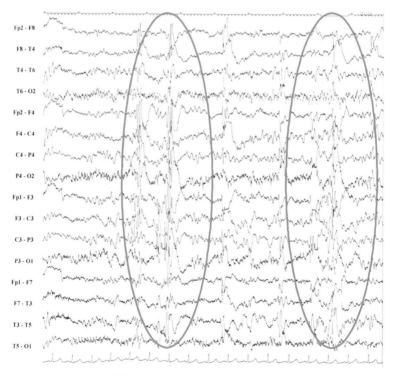

Figure 2.5 Interictal EEG of a patient with juvenile myoclonic epilepsy showing generalized, multiple spike-and-wave complexes (circled).

The AED of choice is VPA. Other useful drugs include lamotrigine (LTG), topiramate (TPM), zonisamide (ZNS) and levetiracetam (LEV). Phenytoin (PHT), CBZ, oxcarbazepine (OXC) and gabapentin (GBP) may exacerbate the myoclonic seizures. The seizures respond well to treatment but usually recur when medication is withdrawn. Therefore, lifelong therapy is generally recommended.

Febrile convulsions develop in association with fever (usually during the rapidly rising phase) with no evidence of another defined cause. They typically present between the ages of 3 months and 5 years. There may be a family history of epilepsy. The incidence is approximately 4%. Up to 1 in 3 affected children will have recurrent febrile seizures. Although febrile seizures are generally benign, around 5% of children with febrile convulsions later develop epilepsy.

Poor prognostic factors include seizures that have focal features or that last longer than 15 minutes, focal neurological abnormalities and a family history of afebrile seizures. Some children will go on to develop mesial temporal sclerosis and partial seizures that are often refractory to AED therapy.

Treatment of febrile convulsions is usually symptomatic, with sponge bathing and prompt administration of an antipyretic. Some physicians advocate prophylactic rectal diazepam for fever in children who have a previous history of febrile convulsions. Most pediatric neurologists would not recommend long-term AED treatment for children with simple febrile seizures (i.e. generalized seizures lasting less than 15 minutes).

Infantile spasms are sudden, brief seizures that are typically tonic flexor spasms of the waist, extremities and neck. They are usually seen as part of West syndrome, which is defined as infantile spasms, hypsarrhythmic patterns on the EEG and severe encephalopathy with psychomotor retardation.

Infantile spasms are associated with 20% mortality; death usually results from the underlying pathology. Of the infants who survive, more than 75% are mentally retarded and more than 50% continue to have seizures throughout life.

Etiology may be known, for example cerebral malformations (half of all patients with tuberous sclerosis develop infantile spasms), perinatal brain damage and postnatal cerebral insults, or it may be idiopathic. Spasms typically begin before 12 months of age, with peak onset at 4 to 6 months of age. Seizures may occur dozens, if not hundreds, of times daily. In addition to massive flexor spasms, abduction or adduction of the arms, self-hugging movements and extensor contractions of the neck and trunk may be seen.

The EEG is markedly abnormal in the majority of cases and consists of diffuse high-voltage spikes and slow waves superimposed on a disorganized, slow background (hypsarrhythmia).

Infantile spasms are often difficult to control. Traditionally, adrenocorticotropic hormone (ACTH), corticosteroids, VPA and nitrazepam have been used. More recently, vigabatrin (VGB) has demonstrated superior efficacy to steroids and is regarded as the treatment of choice by many pediatric neurologists (see Chapter 5, Antiepileptic drugs).

Lennox–Gastaut syndrome is a devastating disorder in children that consists of mixed types of seizures and mental retardation. The EEG is characterized by slow (less than 2.5 Hz) spike-and-wave patterns superimposed on an abnormal, slow background.

Seizures typically occur daily, often in the tens or hundreds, and consist of axial tonic, tonic–clonic, atypical absence, myoclonic and atonic seizures, which often cause injuries. Brief tonic seizures usually occur during the night, sometimes in clusters. Atonic seizures may vary from head drops to catastrophic falls.

Cognitive deficit is usually present before the seizures develop and may be associated with behavioral problems. Most children demonstrate abnormalities on neurological examination.

Prognosis for seizure remission is poor and response to AED therapy is generally unsatisfactory. Drugs showing some efficacy include VPA, LTG, TPM and felbamate (FBM).

Mesial temporal lobe epilepsy (MTLE). Hippocampal sclerosis (HS) is the most common pathology in intractable temporal lobe epilepsy.

Although not recognized as such in the current international classification, many specialists regard MTLE associated with HS as a discrete syndrome.

Onset of seizures usually occurs before puberty, often with a history of prolonged febrile convulsions in childhood. A seizure typically begins with vegetative auras, such as epigastric rising, or affective symptoms (most commonly fear), but may consist of complex delusional experiences, hallucinations, or olfactory or gustatory sensations. When the complex partial seizure ensues, impairment of consciousness is usually heralded by arrest and stare, followed by oroalimentary, gestural and reactive automatisms lasting 1–2 minutes, which the patient does not remember. Afterwards, the patient is confused for varying periods. Post-ictal dysphasia may occur if the seizure involves the language-dominant hemisphere. Secondary generalization is relatively uncommon.

The diagnosis is supported by anterior temporal interictal spikes on a surface EEG, and hippocampal atrophy and signal change on MRI (Figure 2.6).

The disorder may initially respond well to AED treatment, but patients become drug resistant from early adulthood. However, if appropriately selected, up to 80% of patients with pharmacoresistant epilepsy can be rendered seizure free by anterior temporal lobectomy.

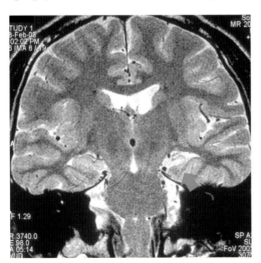

Figure 2.6 MRI scan of a patient with mesial temporal lobe epilepsy showing left hippocampal sclerosis (arrow).

Genetics

Epilepsy is part of the phenotype in more than 200 inherited disorders. Although numerous, genetic syndromes probably account for less than 1% of all cases of epilepsy. They often result in a developmental abnormality, or irreversible and progressive neuronal cell loss in the brain. Therefore, in these conditions, epilepsy is accompanied by other neurological deficits, such as learning disabilities, dementia or ataxia. Examples include a range of inherited metabolic disorders, mitochondrial encephalopathies and neuronal migration disorders.

A small number of inherited epilepsies are 'pure' idiopathic epilepsy syndromes, for which there has been an explosion in molecular understanding over the past 15 years (Table 2.3). Over ten genes have been identified so far, and the number is set to increase in the coming years.

TABLE 2.3

Examples of genes identified in inherited epilepsy syndromes

Syndrome	Gene	Gene product
Benign familial neonatal convulsions	KCNQ2, KCNQ3	Voltage-gated potassium channel subunits
Benign familial neonatal-infantile seizures	SCN2A	Voltage-gated sodium channel, α-2 subunit
Autosomal-dominant nocturnal frontal lobe epilepsy	CHRNA4, CHRAB2	Nicotinic acetylcholine receptor subunits
Autosomal-dominant lateral temporal lobe epilepsy	LGI1	Leucine-rich glioma-inactivated protein
Generalized epilepsy with febrile seizures plus	SCN1A, SCN2A, SCN1B GABRG2	Voltage-gated sodium channel subunits GABA$_A$ receptor, γ-2 subunit
Severe myoclonic epilepsy of infancy	SCN1A	Voltage-gated sodium channel, α-1 subunit

GABA, gamma-aminobutyric acid.

In general, the presumptive causal mutations have been identified in large families with an autosomal-dominant inheritance pattern. Almost all mutations occur in genes that encode voltage-gated or ligand-gated ion channels. How these 'channelopathies' lead to recurrent, episodic seizures remains unclear in most cases.

It has also become apparent that a specific mutation can give rise to a variety of phenotypes or clinical manifestations, and that a single seizure phenotype can be associated with different mutations.

It is important to point out that epilepsy syndromes with Mendelian inheritance are rare. Nevertheless, the discovery of mutations for these rare disorders has provided a foundation for identifying the genetic defects in the more common idiopathic epilepsy syndromes, such as childhood absence epilepsy and JME, which have complex inheritance and likely polygenic involvement.

Key points – classification of seizures and syndromes

- A seizure is a symptom of brain dysfunction.
- Depending on the pattern of onset, seizures are broadly classified into partial and generalized types; classification has important implications for prognosis and management.
- Epileptic syndromes are defined by clinical features, aided by appropriate investigations, including electroencephalography and brain imaging.
- Benign rolandic epilepsy occurs in otherwise neurologically normal children, and generally has an excellent response to antiepileptic drugs (AEDs).
- Long-term AED treatment for children with simple febrile seizures is not recommended.
- Mesial temporal lobe epilepsy is often drug resistant but may be successfully treated by temporal lobectomy.
- Genetic mutations of ion channels have been identified in a range of rare idiopathic epilepsy syndromes.

Locating the channel abnormalities that lead to an expression of epilepsy may provide an insight into the mechanisms of excitability and seizure production, not only in genetically predetermined epilepsy but also in acquired types. It is also hoped that pharmacogenomics will provide a range of novel targets for future AED development.

Key references

Camfield P, Camfield C. Epileptic syndromes in childhood: clinical features, outcomes, and treatment. *Epilepsia* 2002;43(suppl 3):27–32.

Commission on Classification and Terminology of the International League Against Epilepsy. Proposal for revised clinical and electroencephalographic classification of epileptic seizures. *Epilepsia* 1981; 22:489–501.

Commission on Classification and Terminology of the International League Against Epilepsy. Proposal for revised classification of epilepsies and epileptic syndromes. *Epilepsia* 1989;30:389–99.

Gutierrez-Delicado E, Serratosa JM. Genetics of the epilepsies. *Curr Opin Neurol* 2004;17:147–53.

King MA, Newton MR, Jackson GD et al. Epileptology of the first-seizure presentation: a clinical, electroencephalographic, and magnetic resonance imaging study of 300 consecutive patients. *Lancet* 1998;352:1007–11.

Mattson RH. Overview: idiopathic generalized epilepsies. *Epilepsia* 2003;44(suppl 2):2–6.

Nabbout R, Dulac O. Epileptic encephalopathies: a brief overview. *J Clin Neurophysiol* 2003;20:393–7.

Prasad AN, Prasad C, Stafstrom CE. Recent advances in the genetics of epilepsy: insights from human and animal studies. *Epilepsia* 1999; 40:1329–52.

Steinlein OK. Genetic mechanisms that underlie epilepsy. *Nat Rev Neurosci* 2004;5:400–8.

Wheless JW, Kim HL. Adolescent seizures and epilepsy syndromes. *Epilepsia* 2002;43(suppl 3):33–52.

The diagnosis of epilepsy relies on the correct classification of epileptic seizures and epilepsy syndromes (see Chapter 2), with consequent implications for prognosis and choice of therapy.

Epilepsy is not a single disease but an extensive collection of conditions with a wide range of underlying etiologies and pathologies, all sharing the common and fundamental characteristic of recurrent, usually unprovoked seizures. Figure 3.1 shows some common etiologies in relation to age.

The diagnostic procedure aims to answer three key questions:
1. Is the episode an epileptic seizure?
2. What is (are) the seizure type(s)?
3. What is the epilepsy syndrome?

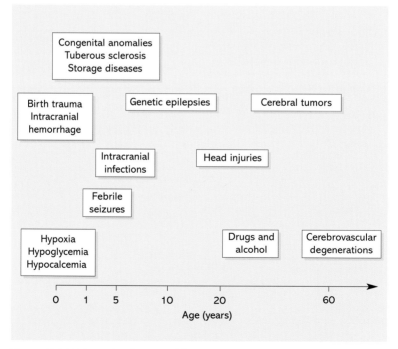

Figure 3.1 Etiology of epilepsy at different ages.

Differential diagnosis

A wide range of conditions can mimic epileptic seizures and must be considered in the differential diagnosis (Table 3.1). For example, syncopal attacks, sometimes with clonic movements and incontinence, are commonly misdiagnosed as epileptic seizures. Furthermore, pseudoseizures or non-epileptic psychogenic seizures are estimated to occur in up to 45% of patients referred to specialist centers with apparently refractory epilepsy. This misidentification of non-epileptic conditions as epilepsy can lead to unnecessary and potentially harmful treatments, and can delay the start of appropriate therapy. The temptation to attach a label of 'epilepsy' should be resisted if there is any doubt about the diagnosis despite a thorough evaluation. Both the physician and patient must simply await the passage of time before coming to a firm conclusion. Further challenges of diagnosis and management may arise in patients in whom non-epileptic attacks coexist with epilepsy or develop as a substitute for seizures once the epilepsy is controlled.

TABLE 3.1

Common differential diagnoses of seizures

Neurological	Endocrine/metabolic
Transient ischemic attack	Hypoglycemia
Transient global amnesia	Hyponatremia
Migraine	Hypokalemia
Narcolepsy	**Sleep disorders**
Cardiac	Obstructive sleep apnea
Vasovagal syncope	Hypnic jerks
Reflex anoxic seizure	Benign neonatal sleep myoclonus
Sick sinus syndrome	REM sleep disorder
Arrhythmias	**Psychological**
Hypotension	Non-epileptic psychogenic seizures

REM, rapid eye movement.

Clinical evaluation

Despite advances in investigational technologies, the diagnosis of epilepsy remains essentially clinical, and is based on a detailed description of the events experienced by the patient before, during and after a seizure. A witness's account of one or more of the episodes is an essential component of a confident diagnosis (Table 3.2). In addition to

TABLE 3.2

Important points in history taking in a patient suspected of having had one or more seizures

Features of the suspected seizure event	Patient's history
Before the event	Previous medical history
– Precipitating or provoking factors	– Birth history
– Preceding symptoms	– Childhood febrile convulsion(s)
– Duration of symptoms	– Severe head trauma or other neurological insult
During the event	– Psychiatric illness
– Motor symptoms	Family history
– Sensory symptoms	Drug history
– Level of awareness/ responsiveness	– Prescribed medication
– Tongue biting or other injury	– Over-the-counter medication
– Urinary incontinence	– Illicit drugs
– Duration of event	– Alcohol use
After the event	
– Level of alertness	
– Confusion	
– Duration of symptoms	
Pattern of events	
– Duration	
– Frequency	
– Stereotyped or variable	

a full medical and social history, the patient should be asked about
factors that may precipitate seizures by lowering the threshold for such
an event (Table 3.3). Physical examination is often unremarkable,
although there may be focal neurological signs that correspond to an
underlying structural abnormality in the brain. Investigations aiming to
unearth any acute provoking cause of seizures should be guided by the
clinical scenario. Routine blood tests should include full blood count
and electrolytes, and an electrocardiogram should be performed to
detect cardiac arrhythmias. Drug screening may be obtained when the
history suggests drug abuse. Lumbar puncture for cerebrospinal fluid
examination should be reserved for those suspected of having an acute
infection of the central nervous system.

Investigational technologies

Electroencephalography can support the clinical diagnosis of epilepsy
and help with the classification of partial-onset or generalized seizures.
It is important to give the electroencephalographer detailed information
concerning the patient's age, seizure behavior and response to
antiepileptic drugs.

TABLE 3.3

Factors lowering seizure threshold

Common	Occasional
Sleep deprivation	Dehydration
Alcohol withdrawal	Barbiturate withdrawal
Television flicker	Benzodiazepine withdrawal
Epileptogenic drugs	Hyperventilation
Systemic infection	Flashing lights
Head trauma	Diet and missed meals
Recreational drugs	Specific 'reflex' triggers
Antiepileptic drug non-compliance	Stress
Menstruation	Intense exercise

Routine electroencephalograms (EEGs) are often insensitive – more than 50% of patients with epilepsy will have a normal trace. Activation techniques, including hyperventilation and photic stimulation (Figure 3.2), are helpful in uncovering abnormalities. Diagnostic yield can also be increased by repeat recordings. If the initial EEG is unremarkable and the diagnosis remains in doubt, a sleep-deprivation study is recommended.

Routine EEGs have a limited role in determining whether a patient may have their AED(s) safely tapered after a prolonged seizure-free interval. In a patient with suspected non-convulsive status epilepticus, an EEG can be diagnostic. An EEG can also immediately differentiate between genuine and 'pseudo' status epilepticus.

Prolonged ambulatory recording. In cases of a negative standard EEG, better detection of interictal and ictal events may be achieved with a prolonged EEG recording using portable equipment. On the plus side, this allows recording to take place in the patient's usual environment, but technical faults are more likely, and accurate

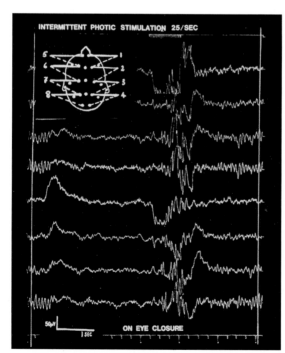

Figure 3.2

Photoconvulsive response provoked by intermittent photic stimulation.

correlation with simultaneous behaviors on video is available only on certain recording systems.

Video-EEG telemetry. Behavioral correlation can be achieved in inpatients by video monitoring during the EEG. This investigation is mandatory as part of the evaluation for epilepsy surgery, and may be the only way to distinguish epileptic from non-epileptic seizures.

Magnetoencephalography has been the subject of recent research, in which the magnetic fields associated with the intracellular current flows within neurons are measured in between seizures. Its usefulness in identifying surgical candidates with normal structural neuroimaging results is under investigation.

Brain imaging

Structural imaging. Imaging studies of the brain to look for underlying structural abnormalities are essential for the appropriate diagnostic evaluation of most patients with epilepsy, particularly those presenting with partial-onset seizures. The imaging modality of choice is magnetic resonance imaging (MRI). It has higher sensitivity and specificity than computed tomography (CT) for identifying structural lesions such as malformations of cortical development (Figure 3.3a), hippocampal sclerosis, arteriovenous malformations, cavernous hemangioma (Figure 3.3b) and low-grade gliomas (Figure 3.3c). CT scanning should be performed if MRI is unavailable, or in patients for whom MRI is contraindicated (e.g. those with cardiac pacemakers, non-compatible aneurysm clips or severe claustrophobia).

Typical pathological findings vary with age. In children, MRI is particularly useful in identifying congenital abnormalities, such as neuronal migration disorders and arteriovenous malformations. In young adulthood, frequently detected conditions are mesial temporal sclerosis, sequelae of head trauma, congenital anomalies, brain tumors and vascular lesions. In mid-life and beyond, scans are helpful in evaluating stroke and cerebral degeneration, and in identifying primary and secondary neoplasia.

Any patient with refractory epilepsy whose initial MRI scan is normal should have a high-resolution scan to exclude hippocampal

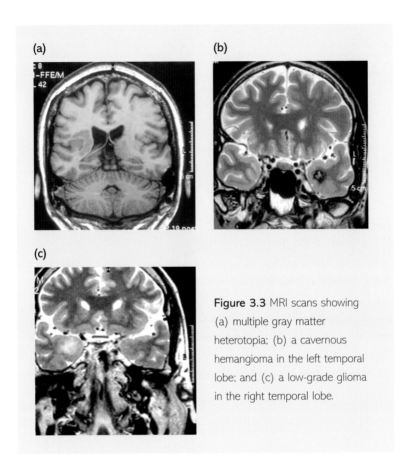

Figure 3.3 MRI scans showing (a) multiple gray matter heterotopia; (b) a cavernous hemangioma in the left temporal lobe; and (c) a low-grade glioma in the right temporal lobe.

atrophy and focal cortical dysplasia. The scan should be repeated periodically if there is one of the following:

- suspicion of a tumor
- worsening in the patient's neurological or cognitive function
- deterioration in the frequency or severity of the seizures.

Functional imaging can identify focal abnormalities in cerebral physiology even when structural imaging results are normal. Single photon emission computed tomography can demonstrate increased blood flow in brain regions associated with seizure activity. Epileptogenic areas can be detected as hypometabolic regions interictally by positron emission tomography (PET) (Figure 3.4). Magnetic resonance spectroscopy can measure changes in chemical

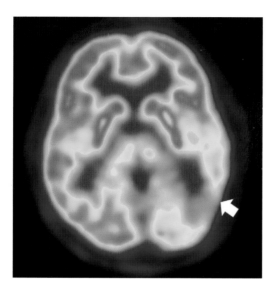

Figure 3.4 PET scan showing interictal hypometabolism over the left temporal and occipital areas.

compounds in the brain associated with neuronal loss in certain epileptogenic pathologies. Functional neuroimaging techniques have a limited role in routine diagnostic evaluation, but are useful adjuncts in the workup for epilepsy surgery.

Key points – diagnosis

- Epilepsy has many underlying etiologies.
- A wide range of conditions can mimic epileptic seizures.
- A witness's account is essential for accurate diagnosis of epilepsy and classification of seizures.
- Electroencephalography can support diagnosis and help with the classification of seizures and syndromes.
- Structural brain imaging is essential in the diagnostic workup for patients with seizures suspected of having a focal onset.
- Magnetic resonance imaging is the imaging modality of choice for detecting structural abnormalities in the brain.
- Functional neuroimaging techniques are mainly used as supplementary investigations in patients being considered for epilepsy surgery.

Key references

Binnie CD, Stefan H. Modern electroencephalography: its role in epilepsy management. *Clin Neurophysiol* 1999;110:1671–97.

Duncan JS. Imaging and epilepsy. *Brain* 1997;120:339–77.

Gilbert DL, Sethuraman G, Kotagal U, Buncher CR. Meta-analysis of EEG test performance shows wide variation among studies. *Neurology* 2003;60:564–70.

Lee BI, Heo K, Kim JS et al. Syndromic diagnosis at the epilepsy clinic: role of MRI in lobar epilepsies. *Epilepsia* 2002;43:496–504.

Manford M. Assessment and investigation of possible epileptic seizures. *J Neurol Neurosurg Psychiatry* 2001;70(suppl 2):II3–8.

Reuber M, Elger CE. Psychogenic nonepileptic seizures: review and update. *Epilepsy Behav* 2003;4: 205–16.

Scottish Intercollegiate Guidelines Network (SIGN). Guideline No. 70. Diagnosis and management of epilepsy in adults. Edinburgh: SIGN, Royal College of Physicians, 2003. www.sign.ac.uk/guidelines/fulltext/ 70/index.html

Smith D, Defalla BA, Chadwick DW. The misdiagnosis of epilepsy and the management of refractory epilepsy in a specialist clinic. *QJM* 1999;92: 15–23.

So EL. Role of neuroimaging in the management of seizure disorders. *Mayo Clin Proc* 2002;77:1251–64.

Starting treatment

Several questions need to be addressed when deciding whether
to prescribe an antiepileptic drug (AED) to a patient presenting
with a seizure.

- What is the chance of recurrence?
- What are the potential negative consequences upon the patient's
  life if seizures recur?
- What are the potential adverse effects of treatment?

After a single seizure. Whether treatment should be started after a
single episode remains controversial. Depending on study methodology
and inclusion criteria, the probability of recurrence over the next
5 years after a single unprovoked seizure ranges from 31% to 71%.
Since a substantial proportion of such patients will not have further
episodes, most specialists do not routinely recommend treatment
after a single seizure. Prospective randomized studies have shown that,
compared with delaying treatment until a further episode, immediate
treatment after a first generalized tonic–clonic seizure does not improve
the long-term remission rate. However, treatment should be considered
after the first seizure when the chance of recurrence is high, for
instance in the presence of an underlying cerebral lesion, an abnormal
electroencephalogram (EEG) or a strong family history of epilepsy,
or if the patient has a high-risk epilepsy syndrome, such as juvenile
myoclonic epilepsy (JME). In some instances, the patient may wish to
start treatment after a single event because they are concerned about
the potential significant impact that recurrent seizures could have upon
their psychosocial functioning, for example their ability to drive.

After more than one seizure. Generally speaking, patients reporting
more than one well-documented or witnessed seizure require treatment.
Exceptions can include widely separated seizures, provoked seizures
for which avoidance activity may be sufficient prophylaxis

(e.g. concomitant illness, photosensitive epilepsy, alcohol withdrawal) and certain benign childhood epilepsy syndromes such as benign rolandic epilepsy. In addition, treatment is unlikely to succeed in patients unlikely or unwilling to take medication (e.g. alcohol abusers, drug addicts, people who refuse to take medication on principle).

An informed choice. The decision whether or not to start treatment should be made after ample discussion with the patient and their family of the risks and benefits of both courses of action. The information should be presented to the patient in the context of what is known and what is conjecture about the risk of recurrent seizures, the chance of a successful outcome with treatment and the likelihood of remission. Pushing the issue if there is doubt about the diagnosis, particularly if the patient resists the introduction of AED therapy, may be counterproductive. Ideally, the patient should be encouraged to make an informed commitment to the treatment plan.

Reasons for taking prophylactic therapy should be discussed at the outset. When prescribing an AED, the clinician must also discuss all common side effects, as well as uncommon but serious side effects such as the risk of teratogenesis in women of childbearing potential. That the latter has been touched upon should be documented in the patient's case notes. Similarly, regulations regarding driving need to be raised and documented. Time should be taken to deal with the patient's fears, misconceptions and prejudices, as well as those of the family. The importance of total compliance with medication should also be stressed. These issues often require further emphasis at subsequent visits. The possibility of sudden unexpected death should be discussed if appropriate, especially if compliance is an issue or if seizures remain uncontrolled (see page 11). The provision of written material can be a useful way to ensure that nothing important has been overlooked.

Principles of drug selection

The goal of treatment should be maintenance of a normal lifestyle by complete seizure control without, or with minimal, side effects. Choosing the most suitable AED for an individual patient requires in-depth knowledge of the characteristics of the epilepsy, the patient and the available AEDs. The issues discussed below should be included in the decision-making process.

Monotherapy. In comparison with combination therapy, monotherapy is associated with better compliance and fewer side effects. It is therefore also likely to be more cost-effective. For these reasons, in general, monotherapy trials of two AEDs that are appropriate first-line treatment for the patient's seizure type(s) should usually be initiated before combinations are tried (Figure 4.1). Since the chance of remission is highest with the first drug – 60% of patients with newly diagnosed epilepsy achieve seizure control with the first or second AED – substantial attention should be given to choosing the most appropriate initial AED.

Efficacy and tolerability. Effectiveness is a function of efficacy and tolerability. Given that lifelong treatment may often be required, even in patients with mild epilepsy, safety and lack of long-term sequelae are important considerations when selecting treatment.

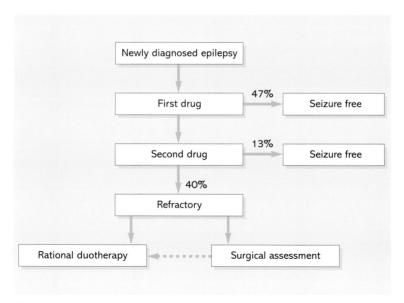

Figure 4.1 Strategies for managing newly diagnosed epilepsy. Data from Kwan et al. 2000.

Titration and monitoring. Approximately 50% of newly diagnosed patients will be able to tolerate and become seizure free with the first AED, often in low or moderate doses. In general, the AED should be started at a low dose, with increments over a number of weeks to establish an effective and tolerable regimen, although some agents, such as gabapentin (GBP) and levetiracetam, can be commenced at effective doses with, or even without, a rapid titration phase. Slow titration will help avoid concentration-dependent side effects, in particular central nervous system toxicity, the presence of which is likely to discourage the patient from persevering with therapy long term. An additional benefit of a cautious approach is that it allows tolerance to develop to sedation or cognitive impairment. Such a policy will also ensure early detection of potentially serious idiosyncratic reactions, such as rash, hepatotoxicity and blood dyscrasias (see Side effects, pages 42–46).

Measuring AED serum concentrations can help to ensure compliance, to assess side effects and to establish the most effective concentration in a seizure-free patient. AED serum concentrations associated with optimal control or with neurotoxicity vary from patient to patient and may occur below, within or above the so-called 'therapeutic' or 'target' ranges for the drugs, particularly in children and in elderly patients. These ranges should be regarded, therefore, purely as a guide to prescribing. Routine measurement of serum levels of the newer AEDs is not otherwise recommended, since they do not correlate well on a population basis with efficacy or side effects.

Measurement of free serum phenytoin (PHT) concentrations can occasionally be useful when patients have low serum albumin levels or take other tightly protein-bound medications. Women who experience an exacerbation of seizures just before their menses should have serum AED concentrations checked in the premenstrual period and compared with mid-cycle concentrations, as levels can drop markedly just before and during menstruation.

If the first drug is well tolerated but the seizures persist, the dose should be increased towards the limit of tolerability, aiming for complete seizure freedom. If the first AED produces an idiosyncratic reaction, side effects at low or moderate doses, or fails to improve seizure control, an alternative should be substituted.

Matching treatment to seizure type. The profile of activity against different seizure types varies among the AEDs (Tables 4.1 and 4.2). Certain epilepsy syndromes have been found to be particularly responsive to specific therapeutic agents. For instance, JME responds well to sodium valproate (VPA), while many pediatricians regard vigabatrin (VGB) as the drug of choice for infantile spasms. On the other hand, myoclonic and absence seizures can be exacerbated by PHT and carbamazepine (CBZ). It is therefore of paramount importance to accurately classify the patient's seizure type(s) and epilepsy syndrome (see Chapter 2). Recommended drug choices for adults and children according to seizure types are shown in Tables 4.3 and 4.4, respectively. The recommendations are based on the current literature and recent UK and US treatment guidelines. Because of the paucity of head-to-head comparative studies, particularly for the newer AEDs, the evidence base is supplemented by the authors' personal experience. It is anticipated that the tables will require updating as new trial data emerge.

TABLE 4.1

Efficacy of established antiepileptic drugs against common seizure types and syndromes

Type of seizure/ syndrome	CBZ	CLB	CZP	ESM	PB	PHT	PRM	VPA
Partial	+	+	+	O	+	+	+	+
Secondary generalized	+	+	+	O	+	+	+	+
Tonic–clonic	+	+	+	O	+	+	+	+
Absence	–	?	?	+	O	–	O	+
Myoclonic	–	+	+	O	?+	–	?	+
Lennox–Gastaut	O	+	?+	O	?	O	?	+
Infantile spasms	O	?+	?+	O	?	O	?	+

+ proven efficacy; ?+ probable efficacy; O ineffective; – worsens control; ? unknown.
CBZ, carbamazepine; CLB, clobazam; CZP, clonazepam; ESM, ethosuximide; PB, phenobarbital; PHT, phenytoin; PRM, primidone; VPA, sodium valproate.

TABLE 4.2

Efficacy of newer antiepileptic drugs against common seizure types and syndromes

Type of seizure/ syndrome	FBM	GBP	LEV	LTG	OXC	PGB	TGB	TPM	VGB	ZNS
Partial	+	+	+	+	+	+	+	+	+	+
Secondary generalized	+	+	+	+	+	+	+	+	+	+
Tonic–clonic	?+	?+	+	+	+	?	?	+	?+	+
Absence	?+	–	?+	+	–	?	–	?	–	?+
Myoclonic	?	–	+	+*	–	?	?	+	–	+
Lennox–Gastaut	+	?	?	+	0	?	?	+	?	?+
Infantile spasms	?	?	?	?+	0	?	?+	?+	+	?+

*Lamotrigine may worsen myoclonic seizures in some cases.
+ proven efficacy; ?+ probable efficacy; 0 ineffective; – worsens control; ? unknown.
FBM, felbamate; GBP, gabapentin; LEV, levetiracetam; LTG, lamotrigine; OXC, oxcarbazepine; PGB, pregabalin; TGB, tiagabine; TPM, topiramate; VGB, vigabatrin; ZNS, zonisamide.

For partial seizures and generalized tonic–clonic seizures (the most common seizure types), the established AEDs, with the exception of ethosuximide (ESM), appear to have similar efficacy. There is a possible small benefit of CBZ over VPA for partial seizures. Phenobarbital (PB) has demonstrated higher withdrawal rates due to its sedative effect.

None of the newer AEDs has shown superior efficacy when tested against the established agents for the treatment of partial seizures and generalized tonic–clonic seizures, but some have demonstrated better tolerability, in particular fewer neurotoxic side effects (Table 4.5). Thus, lamotrigine (LTG) and oxcarbazepine (OXC) showed better overall effectiveness than did CBZ and PHT, respectively.

Side effects. Safety concerns include idiosyncratic reactions, long-term complications and teratogenicity. The most common idiosyncratic

TABLE 4.3

Choice of antiepileptic drugs in adolescents and adults according to seizure type*

Seizure type	First line	Second line/ add-on	Third line/ add-on
Absence (typical and atypical)	VPA LTG	ESM	LEV ZNS
Myoclonic	VPA	TPM LEV ZNS	LTG CLB CZP PB
Tonic–clonic	VPA CBZ PHT PB†	LTG OXC	TPM LEV ZNS PRM
Atonic	VPA	LTG TPM	FBM
Simple and complex partial, with or without secondary generalization	CBZ PHT PB† OXC LTG TPM GBP	VPA LEV ZNS PGB	TGB VGB FBM PRM
Unclassifiable	VPA	LTG	TPM LEV ZNS

*Other selection criteria include patient characteristics, side-effect profile, potential drug–drug interactions, availability and cost (see text).
†Phenobarbital is often regarded as second-line therapy because of sedation and behavioral problems.
CBZ, carbamazepine; CLB, clobazam; CZP, clonazepam; ESM, ethosuximide; FBM, felbamate; GBP, gabapentin; LEV, levetiracetam; LTG, lamotrigine; OXC, oxcarbazepine; PB, phenobarbital; PGB, pregabalin; PHT, phenytoin; PRM, primidone; TGB, tiagabine; TPM, topiramate; VGB, vigabatrin; VPA, sodium valproate; ZNS, zonisamide.

reaction to AEDs is skin rash, which can range from a trivial evanescent exanthema to a life-threatening Stevens–Johnson syndrome or toxic epidermal necrolysis. The association of felbamate (FBM) with

43

TABLE 4.4

Choice of antiepileptic drugs in children according to seizure type*

Seizure type	First line	Second line/ add-on	Third line/ add-on
Absence (typical and atypical)	VPA LTG	ESM	CLB ZNS
Myoclonic	VPA	TPM ZNS	LTG CLB PB
Tonic–clonic	VPA CBZ PB†	LTG TPM PHT	ZNS OXC LEV
Simple and complex partial, with or without secondary generalization	CBZ VPA PB†	LTG TPM OXC ZNS	CLB PHT GBP‡ LEV
Infantile spasms	VGB ACTH	VPA NTZ	LTG ZNS TPM
Lennox–Gastaut	VPA	LTG TPM	CLB FBM
Unclassifiable	VPA	LTG	TPM LEV ZNS

*Other selection criteria include patient characteristics, side-effect profile, potential drug–drug interactions, availability and cost (see text).
†Phenobarbital is often regarded as second-line therapy because of sedation and behavioral problems. It is restricted for use in neonates in many developed countries.
‡Not approved for use in the pediatric population.
ACTH, adrenocorticotropic hormone; CBZ, carbamazepine; CLB, clobazam; ESM, ethosuximide; FBM, felbamate; GBP, gabapentin; LEV, levetiracetam; LTG, lamotrigine; NTZ, nitrazepam; OXC, oxcarbazepine; PB, phenobarbital; PHT, phenytoin; TPM, topiramate; VGB, vigabatrin; VPA, sodium valproate; ZNS, zonisamide.

aplastic anemia and hepatotoxicity has relegated it to the drug of last choice. Rare cases of acute glaucoma and clinically important hypohydrosis have been reported with topiramate (TPM).

TABLE 4.5

Adverse effects of antiepileptic drugs (AEDs) on cognition and behavior

AED	Cognitive	Behavioral
Established AEDs		
Carbamazepine	+	0
Clobazam	+	+
Clonazepam	++	+
Ethosuximide	+	+
Phenobarbital	++	++
Phenytoin	+	0
Primidone	++	++
Sodium valproate	+	0
Newer AEDs		
Felbamate	0	+
Gabapentin	0	0
Lamotrigine	0	0
Levetiracetam	0	+
Oxcarbazepine	+?	0
Pregabalin	0	0
Tiagabine	0	0
Topiramate	+*	+?
Vigabatrin	0	+
Zonisamide	0	+?

*Risk reduced by slow titration.
0 no effect; +? possible effect; + mild effect; ++ marked effect.

Long-term use of some AEDs can lead to dysmorphic changes, such as gum hypertrophy with PHT, and weight gain with VPA and, to a lesser extent, GBP and pregabalin (PGB). VPA can also be associated with polycystic ovaries and hyperinsulinemia in susceptible women. Among the newer AEDs, the high incidence of concentric visual field defects in patients receiving VGB has substantially reduced the clinical use of this otherwise effective agent. Certain AEDs, such as PB, TPM and VGB are more commonly associated with neuropsychiatric complications and should be used cautiously in patients with a history of mental illness.

The established AEDs have all been shown to increase the likelihood of fetal malformation. Recent analysis from several large-scale prospective registries suggests that the risk of major malformation may be particularly high with VPA compared with other established agents. Data regarding the newer AEDs are accumulating, and the teratogenic risk associated with LTG appears to be lower than with CBZ. However, the combination of VPA with LTG may be particularly teratogenic.

Pharmacokinetics and drug–drug interactions. An ideal AED should demonstrate complete absorption, linear kinetics and a long elimination half-life, allowing once- or twice-daily dosing. Low protein binding, lack of active metabolites and clearance by the renal route can also be regarded as advantageous, since such a drug is likely to be easy to use and less likely to be implicated in pharmacokinetic interactions. However, the dosage for drugs that are excreted unchanged by the kidney, such as GBP and PGB, will need to be adjusted in patients with renal impairment in relation to creatinine clearance.

Older AEDs are notorious for their ability to produce pharmacokinetic interactions among themselves as well as with other medications via their effect on the hepatic cytochrome P450 (CYP) enzyme system (Table 4.6). PB, primidone (PRM), PHT and CBZ induce CYP enzymes that accelerate the breakdown of many commonly prescribed lipid-soluble drugs metabolized by the same system, including oral contraceptives, cytotoxics, antiarrhythmics and warfarin. VPA is a weak CYP enzyme inhibitor, which can slow the clearance of other AEDs, such as PHT and LTG. AEDs can also be targets for drugs that induce or inhibit hepatic metabolism. The newer AEDs are less likely to interfere with hepatic metabolism, although OXC, FBM and TPM (at daily doses above 200 mg) selectively induce the breakdown of the estrogenic component of the oral contraceptive pill.

TABLE 4.6

Pharmacokinetic characteristics of antiepileptic drugs (AEDs)

AED	Undergoes hepatic metabolism	Affects drug-metabolizing enzymes	Associated with AED interactions
Established AEDs			
Carbamazepine	Yes	Yes	Yes
Clobazam	Yes	No	Yes
Clonazepam	Yes	No	Yes
Ethosuximide	Yes	No	Yes
Phenobarbital	Yes	Yes	Yes
Phenytoin	Yes	Yes	Yes
Primidone	Yes	Yes	Yes
Sodium valproate	Yes	Yes	Yes
Newer AEDs			
Felbamate	Yes	Yes	Yes
Gabapentin	No	No	No
Lamotrigine	Yes	No	Yes
Levetiracetam	No	No	No
Oxcarbazepine	Yes	Yes	Yes
Pregabalin	No	No	No
Tiagabine	Yes	No	Yes
Topiramate	Yes	Yes	Yes
Vigabatrin	No	No	Yes
Zonisamide	Yes	Yes	Yes

Comorbidities. As well as controlling seizures, some AEDs have demonstrated efficacy for the treatment of other conditions that may coexist with epilepsy. For instance, VPA has traditionally been used in bipolar affective disorder. It is also effective prophylaxis for migraine, an indication for which TPM has also recently been approved. GBP is effective for the treatment of certain neuropathic pain syndromes, while

PGB has demonstrated efficacy for neuropathic pain and generalized anxiety disorder. With a widening spectrum of indications, AED selection may be tailored according to the patient's neurological and psychiatric comorbidities (see Chapter 9, Quality of life).

Bone health. Long-term AED therapy can lead to hypocalcemia and decrease biologically active vitamin D levels, resulting in reduced bone mineral density and higher risk of fractures in patients with epilepsy. Most of the available data pertain to the older drugs, but information regarding newer agents is emerging. Both enzyme-inducing and non-enzyme-inducing agents are implicated, and the effects may be additive. A variety of mechanisms for AED-induced osteoporosis have been suggested, the most important of which appears to be an increased rate of bone turnover. Bone loss can be detected by dual-energy X-ray absorptiometry (DEXA) or quantitative ultrasound.

To reduce the risk of osteoporosis, patients taking long-term AED therapy are advised to maintain the optimal level of physical activity and a balanced diet. They should be advised against smoking and excessive intake of alcohol or caffeine, all of which can exacerbate bone loss. Risk factors for osteoporosis include:

- prolonged therapy
- exposure to multiple drugs
- a non-ambulatory lifestyle
- concomitant steroid therapy.

People at risk are advised to take calcium and vitamin D supplements and undergo regular DEXA scanning. Once osteopenia or osteoporosis has developed, the patient should be referred to an endocrinologist for consideration of bisphosphonate therapy or high-dose vitamin D treatment.

Combination therapy can be considered if monotherapy attempts with first-line AEDs are ineffective, since the chance of successful seizure control with a third choice of monotherapy is slim. If the first AED produces a good response but complete seizure freedom remains elusive, adding a drug with a different mechanism of action may be a more pragmatic strategy in some patients than substitution. Some patients show useful improvement in seizure frequency or severity with a combination of AEDs.

The number of possible two-drug regimens is growing rapidly. Whether it is possible to combine AEDs 'rationally' is being hotly debated. There is some evidence that combinations involving a sodium channel blocker and a drug that facilitates the inhibition of gamma-aminobutyric acid or a drug with multiple mechanisms of action appear to be particularly beneficial. For instance, evidence supporting the beneficial effects of VPA with LTG is mounting. Some useful examples are listed in Table 4.7.

The practical difficulty with combination therapy is that troublesome or disabling side effects are common at high doses, and complex pharmacokinetic interactions can occur. Consequently, combinations of drugs with different side-effect profiles and those that do not have the potential for deleterious drug interactions are advisable. Practical guidelines for prescribing AEDs are summarized in Table 4.8.

Refractory epilepsy

For practical purposes, refractory epilepsy can be suspected when seizure control is not achieved with the first two appropriate and well-tolerated AED schedules taken as monotherapy or in combination. Work-up for epilepsy surgery can be considered at this point,

TABLE 4.7

Combinations of drugs reported to be useful in refractory epilepsy

Combination	Indication
Sodium valproate and ethosuximide	Generalized absences
Carbamazepine and sodium valproate	Complex partial seizures
Sodium valproate and lamotrigine	Partial/generalized seizures
Topiramate and lamotrigine	Partial/generalized seizures
Vigabatrin* and lamotrigine	Partial seizures
Vigabatrin* and tiagabine	Partial seizures

*Because of the high incidence of visual field defects, vigabatrin should be reserved for patients in whom other antiepileptic drugs have failed.

TABLE 4.8

Ten commandments in the pharmacological treatment of epilepsy

- Choose the correct drug for the seizure type and/or epilepsy syndrome
- Start at low dose
- Titrate up slowly to allow development of tolerance to central nervous system side effects
- Keep the regimen simple with once- or twice-daily dosing, if possible
- Measure drug concentration when seizures are controlled or if control is not readily obtained (if possible)
- Counsel the patient early regarding the implications of the diagnosis and the prophylactic nature of drug therapy
- Try two reasonable monotherapy options before adding a second drug in combination therapy
- When seizures persist, combine the best-tolerated first-line drug with one of the newer agents depending on seizure type and mechanism of action
- Simplify dosage schedules and drug regimens as much as possible in patients receiving polypharmacy
- Aim for the best seizure control consistent with optimal quality of life in patients with refractory epilepsy

particularly if a potentially operable structural abnormality, such as mesial temporal sclerosis, has been identified. This is also a good time to evaluate whether there may be any factor responsible for a state of 'pseudoresistance' (Table 4.9), by reviewing:

- security of the diagnosis
- accuracy of the seizure and/or syndrome classification
- results of brain imaging
- the patient's compliance with medication
- the presence of negative lifestyle factors such as covert alcohol or drug abuse.

If the first AED combination is not effective and epilepsy surgery is not an option, a sequence of drug combinations with potential complementary modes of action could be tried. Data to guide further pharmacological management are lacking. A small proportion of patients will become seizure free with three AEDs, but treatment with four or more is highly unlikely to be successful; as the drug burden increases, polytherapy is less likely to be tolerated and therefore is unlikely to be effective. Drug burden is a function of dose as well as numbers, so further introductions may be made possible by reducing the dose of one or more AEDs.

Therapy withdrawal

Successful treatment outcome can be regarded as freedom from seizures without side effects. Such individuals are more likely to lead rewarding lives – with optimal intellectual and emotional development, and positive educational and vocational achievements – than patients with uncontrolled seizures. In short, they will have a better chance of fulfilling their potential. Eventually, many patients can have their medication withdrawn and remain in remission.

TABLE 4.9

Some reasons for 'pseudoresistance' to antiepileptic drug therapy

Wrong diagnosis
Syncope, cardiac arrhythmia, etc.
Malingering, pseudoseizures
Underlying brain neoplasm

Wrong drug(s)
Inappropriate for seizure type
Kinetic/dynamic interactions

Wrong dose
Too low (ignore target range)
Side effects preventing dose increase

Wrong patient
Poor compliance with medication
Inappropriate lifestyle (e.g. alcohol or drug abuse)

Patients who are 'doing well' may want to stop treatment for a variety of reasons, including the awareness of side effects or the subjective perception of subtle deterioration in cognitive function. In addition, some patients do not equate taking medication with normal health. Finally, the patient may want to start a family and may be concerned about the possible negative effects of AEDs on reproductive function, along with the specter of teratogenesis.

Several studies have shown that, after a long period of perfect seizure control, medication can be stopped without seizure recurrence (for several years at least) in around 60% of patients. There are no data to indicate an optimum length for the seizure-free period. In children, 2 years is reasonable, while in adults a flexible 5 years may be more prudent.

Seizure type or epilepsy syndrome is not absolutely predictive of recurrence. However, a few specific childhood syndromes, such as benign rolandic epilepsy and benign familial neonatal convulsions, tend to do well after drug withdrawal, whereas JME conveys a high probability of relapse. Some forms of idiopathic generalized seizures, either absence or tonic–clonic, are less likely to recur once they are under control. Even complex partial seizures can disappear after a long period of freedom from seizures.

The highest probability of remaining seizure free can be seen in patients with the following characteristics:
- relatively few seizures before and after starting AED therapy
- treated with a single AED
- seizure free for many years
- normal neurological examination finding and no structural lesion on brain imaging.

The EEG is not a huge help in predicting seizure recurrence, but a normal investigation is reassuring.

There are no standard protocols defining optimal regimens for tapering medication. Most specialists advise slow reduction by increments over at least 6 months. If the patient is taking two AEDs, one drug should be slowly withdrawn before the second is tapered. More than 90% of recurrences will occur during the year following withdrawal, and many will present during the tapering period or shortly after.

Referral to a specialist

The primary goal of epilepsy management is to restore the patient's functional capacity to its maximal potential. Attaining this goal is often a team effort involving medical and social service professionals and the patient's family, friends and coworkers. The role of the primary care provider varies according to the clinical setting, his/her experience and the patient's needs.

Primary care physicians must be familiar with all the diagnostic and therapeutic options, because they will usually perform the initial evaluation of the first seizure, primarily to exclude non-epileptic causes such as syncope and hypoglycemia. Even experienced primary care physicians may not feel qualified, however, to assume full responsibility for the diagnosis, planning and follow-up of patients with epilepsy. Often, they do not have direct access to the necessary investigational techniques. If a non-epileptic cause of the symptoms is ruled out, the patient should see a neurologist or other appropriate specialist for further diagnostic studies, to determine the likelihood of further seizures and to consider the need for, and choice of, AED therapy. Dose adjustments can be undertaken later by the primary care physician.

The patient should be referred back to the epilepsy specialist if they are:
- unresponsive to treatment with the first two AED schedules
- having significant side effects with treatment
- planning a pregnancy
- considering withdrawal of therapy.

Attending to the patient's psychosocial, cognitive, educational and vocational needs is an important part of caring for people with epilepsy. Both the primary care physician and the epilepsy specialist should work closely with other medical and social service professionals, and extend their roles beyond that of clinician to patient educator and advocate. Subsequent referral to a comprehensive epilepsy center for EEG monitoring, investigational drugs or devices, or consideration of epilepsy surgery is indicated for compliant patients whose seizures prove refractory to two or three reasonable attempts at pharmacological manipulation using new and established AEDs singly and in combination.

Key points – pharmacological management

- Patients reporting more than one unprovoked seizure usually require treatment; treatment after a single unprovoked seizure could be considered if the chance of recurrence is high.
- At the start of treatment, a single antiepileptic drug (AED) should be given and slowly titrated up to a target dosage.
- First-line AEDs should be chosen according to the patient's seizure type(s) and/or epilepsy syndrome. Other important factors include efficacy, safety and lack of long-term sequelae, and a low risk of pharmacokinetic interactions.
- Combination AED therapy could be used after failure of two monotherapies.
- Calcium and vitamin D supplements are recommended for high-risk patients receiving long-term AED treatment.
- None of the newer AEDs has shown superior efficacy when tested against established agents for the treatment of partial seizures and generalized tonic–clonic seizures.
- Patients should be referred to a specialist for definitive diagnosis and initiation of treatment, or when refractory to medication, planning for pregnancy or wanting to withdraw treatment in the case of remission.
- The primary care physician plays an important role in coordinating professional care for people with epilepsy.

Key references

Arroyo S, de la Morena A. Life-threatening adverse events of antiepileptic drugs. *Epilepsy Res* 2001;47:155–74.

Berg AT, Shinnar S. The risk of seizure recurrence following a first unprovoked seizure: a quantitative review. *Neurology* 1991;41:965–72.

Berg AT, Shinnar S. Relapse following discontinuation of antiepileptic drugs: a meta-analysis. *Neurology* 1994;44:601–8.

Brodie MJ, French JA. Management of epilepsy in adolescents and adults. *Lancet* 2000;356:323–9.

Brodie MJ, Kwan P. Staged approach to epilepsy management. *Neurology* 2002;58(8 suppl 5):S2–8.

Deckers CL, Czuczwar SJ, Hekster YA et al. Selection of antiepileptic drug polytherapy based on mechanisms of action: the evidence reviewed. *Epilepsia* 2000;41: 1364–74.

Farhat G, Yamout B, Mikati MA et al. Effect of antiepileptic drugs on bone density in ambulatory patients. *Neurology* 2002;58:1348–53.

Kwan P, Brodie MJ. Early identification of refractory epilepsy. *N Engl J Med* 2000;342:314–19.

Kwan P, Brodie MJ. Effectiveness of first antiepileptic drug. *Epilepsia* 2001;42:1255–60.

Kwan P, Brodie MJ. Neuropsychological effects of epilepsy and antiepileptic drugs. *Lancet* 2001;357:216–22.

Kwan P, Brodie MJ. Clinical trials of antiepileptic medications in newly diagnosed patients with epilepsy. *Neurology* 2003;60(11 suppl 4): S2–12.

Marson A, Jacoby A, Johnson A et al. Immediate versus deferred antiepileptic drug treatment for early epilepsy and single seizures: a randomised controlled trial. *Lancet* 2005;365:2007–13.

Patsalos PN, Fröscher W, Pisani F, van Rijn CM. The importance of drug interactions in epilepsy therapy. *Epilepsia* 2002;43:365–85.

Established antiepileptic drugs

Despite the recent entry into the marketplace of a wide range of new pharmacological options, most patients still receive treatment with one of the established antiepileptic drugs (AEDs). Comparative pharmacokinetics, indications and a guide to dosing in children and adults are summarized in Tables 5.1–5.3.

TABLE 5.1

Pharmacological properties of established antiepileptic drugs

Drug	Primary mode(s) of action	Indications (seizure type)	Absorption (bioavailability %)
Carbamazepine	Sodium channel blockade	Partial, GTCS	Slow (75–80)
Clobazam	GABAergic	Partial, generalized	Rapid (90–100)
Clonazepam	GABAergic	Partial, generalized	Rapid (80–90)
Ethosuximide	Calcium channel blockade	Absence	Rapid (90–95)
Phenobarbital	GABAergic	Partial, GTCS, myoclonic, tonic, clonic, SE	Slow (95–100)
Phenytoin	Sodium channel blockade	Partial, GTCS, SE	Slow (85–90)
Primidone	GABAergic	Partial, GTCS	Rapid (90–100)
Sodium valproate	Multiple	Partial, generalized	Rapid (100)

GABA, gamma-aminobutyric acid; GTCS, generalized tonic–clonic seizures;

In chapter 4 we set out the main principles of drug selection and overall pharmacological management. Here, we consider the use of each drug in terms of its mechanism of action, indication, dosage, tolerability, pharmacokinetics and drug–drug interactions, and highlight problems likely to be encountered in everyday clinical practice.

Carbamazepine (CBZ) was synthesized by Schindler at Geigy in 1953 in an attempt to compete with the newly introduced antipsychotic chlorpromazine. The first clinical studies in epilepsy were not carried

Protein binding (% bound)	Elimination half-life (hours)	Routes of elimination	Target serum concentration
70–80	24–45 (single) 8–24 (chronic)	Hepatic metabolism Active metabolite	4–12 mg/L (17–50 μmol/L)
87–90	10–30	Hepatic metabolism Active metabolite	None
80–90	17–56	Hepatic metabolism	None
0	20–60	Hepatic metabolism 25% excreted unchanged	40–100 mg/L (283–706 μmol/L)
48–54	72–144	Hepatic metabolism 25% excreted unchanged	10–40 mg/L (40–172 μmol/L)
90–93	9–40	Saturable hepatic metabolism	10–20 mg/L (40–80 μmol/L)
20–30	4–12	Hepatic metabolism Active metabolites 40% excreted unchanged	8–12 mg/L (25–50 μmol/L)
88–92	7–17	Hepatic metabolism Active metabolite	50–100 mg/L (350–700 μmol/L)

SE, status epilepticus.

out until 1963. CBZ acts by preventing repetitive firing of action potentials in depolarized neurons via use- and voltage-dependent blockade of sodium channels.

TABLE 5.2

Dosing guidelines for established antiepileptic drugs in adults

Drug	Starting dose (mg/day)	Commonest dose (mg/day)	Maintenance dose (mg/day)	Dosing interval
Carbamazepine	200	600	400–2000	bd–qds
Clobazam	10	20	10–40	od–bd
Clonazepam	1	4	2–8	od–bd
Ethosuximide	500	1000	500–2000	od–bd
Phenobarbital	60	120	60–240	od–bd
Phenytoin	200	300	100–700	od–bd
Primidone	125	500	250–1500	od–bd
Sodium valproate	500	1000	500–3000	bd–tds

od, once daily; bd, twice daily; tds, three times a day; qds, four times a day.

TABLE 5.3

Dosing guidelines for established antiepileptic drugs in children

Drug	Starting dose (mg/kg/day)	Maintenance dose (mg/kg/day)	Dosing interval
Carbamazepine	5	10–25	bd–qds
Clobazam	0.25	0.5–1	od–bd
Clonazepam	0.025	0.025–0.1	bd–tds
Ethosuximide	10	15–30	od–bd
Phenobarbital	4	4–8	od–bd
Phenytoin	5	5–15	od–bd
Primidone	10	20–30	od–bd
Sodium valproate	10	15–40	bd–tds

od, once daily; bd, twice daily; tds, three times a day; qds, four times a day.

Indications. Over the years, CBZ has gained acceptance as a first-line treatment for partial and tonic–clonic seizures. It is not effective, and may even be deleterious, for generalized absences and myoclonic seizures.

Dosage. CBZ should be introduced in low doses (100–200 mg daily) with 100–200 mg increments every 3–14 days, depending on the urgency of the situation. Slow introduction facilitates tolerance to its central nervous system (CNS) side effects and allows hepatic auto-induction of CBZ metabolism to take place. The dose can be increased over the first month or two to a maintenance amount that completely controls the seizure disorder. A balance must be achieved in the individual patient between speed of seizure control and acceptance of temporary CNS toxicity. The final dose will depend on the extent to which CBZ induces its own metabolism (Figure 5.1).

Despite this careful approach, some patients will be unable to tolerate the neurotoxic side effects of CBZ, even at low doses and serum concentrations. Diplopia, headache, dizziness, nausea and vomiting are the most common complaints. For some patients with refractory epilepsy, these symptoms provide a dose ceiling, which may be less than an effective dose. High peak concentrations often result in intermittent side effects around 2 hours after dosing, necessitating administration three or four times daily in some patients. Such problems can be overcome by prescribing a controlled-release formulation that can be

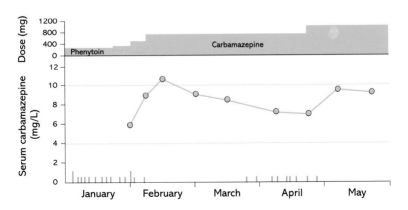

Figure 5.1 Auto-induction of carbamazepine metabolism. The lines at the bottom of the graph represent partial (short) and tonic–clonic (longer) seizures.

given twice daily, or by shifting a greater percentage of the total daily dose to bedtime, particularly when the patient has only nocturnal or early morning seizures.

Side effects. In addition to the CNS toxicity described above, CBZ can cause a range of idiosyncratic reactions, the most common of which is a morbilliform rash in around 10% of patients (Figure 5.2). Other unusual, but more severe, skin eruptions include erythema multiforme and Stevens–Johnson syndrome. Reversible mild leukopenia often occurs within the first few months of treatment, but therapy does not need to be discontinued unless the leukopenia is accompanied by evidence of infection or if the white-cell count slips well below 2000×10^9/liter. Potentially fatal blood dyscrasias and toxic hepatitis are much rarer problems. At high concentrations, the drug has an antidiuretic hormone-like action that can result in fluid retention in patients with cardiac failure and in the elderly. Mild hyponatremia is usually asymptomatic, but if the serum sodium level falls below 120 mmol/liter the patient may present with confusion, peripheral edema and deterioration in seizure control. CBZ is teratogenic. In particular, it is associated with an incidence of around 0.5% of spina bifida in exposed fetuses.

Pharmacokinetics and drug–drug interactions. As well as inducing its own metabolism, CBZ can accelerate the hepatic breakdown of a number of lipid-soluble drugs. The most common interaction is with the oral contraceptive pill, necessitating a daily estrogen dose of 50 µg or more for most women. Other important targets include sodium

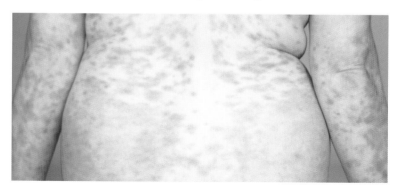

Figure 5.2 Typical morbilliform rash due to carbamazepine.

valproate (VPA), ethosuximide (ESM), corticosteroids, anticoagulants, antipsychotics and ciclosporin.

Drugs that inhibit CBZ metabolism resulting in toxicity include phenytoin (PHT), cimetidine, dextropropoxyphene, diltiazem, erythromycin, isoniazid, verapamil, viloxazine and fluoxetine. The substantial variation in any given patient in CBZ concentrations over the course of a day – as much as 100% with twice-daily dosing – makes the interpretation of concentration monitoring problematic unless the times of dosing and blood sampling are standardized. In many patients, the dose can be titrated adequately on clinical criteria alone. Exceptions include patients suspected of poor compliance and those taking a cocktail of AEDs that are likely to interact with one another.

Phenytoin (PHT). The discovery and clinical testing of PHT by Merritt and Putnam in the 1930s introduced both a major new non-sedating AED and an animal model of epilepsy (electrical seizures in the cat). Like CBZ, PHT blocks voltage-dependent neuronal sodium channels.

Indications. For the past 70 years, PHT has been a first-line medication for the prevention of partial and tonic–clonic seizures and for the acute treatment of seizures and status epilepticus (SE), although it is more often used as a second-line agent in children. PHT is not effective against myoclonic, atonic and absence seizures. It is available in oral and intravenous forms.

Dosage. Depending on the urgency of the situation, PHT may be started at the maintenance dose, typically 300 mg/day as a single dose or in two divided doses in adults (5–8 mg/kg/day in children), or at a higher dose, such as 20 mg/kg divided into three oral doses over 24 hours or 20 mg/kg given intravenously – no faster than 50 mg/minute. The dose should be increased at 1–2 weekly increments as necessary and as tolerated. Most adults usually achieve satisfactory seizure control with once-daily dosing. Patients with erratic compliance should be treated twice daily to lessen the effect of a missed dose.

Side effects can be divided into neurotoxic symptoms (ataxia, nystagmus, dysarthria, asterixis, somnolence) that typically present 8–12 hours after an oral dose, chronic dysmorphic effects (gingival hyperplasia, hirsutism, acne, facial coarsening) that occur after months of therapy, and uncommon, long-term problems (folate deficiency, osteopenia, peripheral neuropathy, cerebellar atrophy) that take years to develop. PHT is associated with rash in approximately 5% of patients. Other rare idiosyncratic reactions include Stevens–Johnson syndrome, hepatitis, bone marrow suppression, lymphadenopathy and a lupus-like syndrome. PHT is also a teratogen.

Pharmacokinetics and drug–drug interactions. PHT is metabolized in the liver. The first step of this process involves the enzyme arene oxidase, which has saturable kinetics, particularly at moderate-to-high serum concentrations. The concentration at which PHT pharmaco-kinetics become non-linear varies as a function of age. As a consequence of this pharmacokinetic profile, small changes in dosing may result in disproportionate changes in serum concentration (Figure 5.3). In all patients, the dose should be increased or decreased by 25–50 mg increments when clinically indicated, particularly when serum concentrations exceed 10 mg/liter. Serum concentrations should then be checked 1–2 weeks later.

PHT induces hepatic enzymes and may, therefore, reduce serum concentrations of metabolized AEDs such as CBZ, VPA, lamotrigine (LTG) and topiramate (TPM). The effectiveness of other lipid-soluble

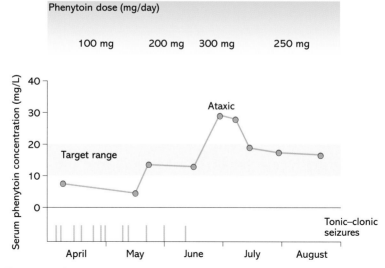

Figure 5.3 Saturation kinetics with phenytoin.

drugs, including oral contraceptives and anticoagulants, is also jeopardized. PHT is tightly bound to circulating albumin and may be displaced by other drugs, some of which, like VPA, also inhibit its metabolism. Checking free PHT serum concentrations may be useful clinically to correlate with a patient's possible neurotoxic symptoms in the setting of hypoalbuminemia, renal and hepatic insufficiency, or pregnancy. Febrile illness may increase the clearance of PHT, resulting in lowered serum concentrations. Enteral feeding has been reported to decrease PHT absorption.

Fosphenytoin is a phosphate ester prodrug of PHT that can be administered intravenously or intramuscularly. It is water soluble and can be given more rapidly with fewer local side effects than intravenous PHT. Although more expensive, fosphenytoin is better tolerated than parenteral PHT and is replacing the latter in the routine treatment of SE.

Sodium valproate (VPA). VPA's anticonvulsant property was recognized serendipitously in 1963, when it was used by Pierre Eymard as a solvent for a number of other compounds. VPA exerts its antiepileptic property, at least in part, by limiting sustained repetitive firing by a use- and voltage-dependent effect on sodium channels. It also facilitates the effects of the inhibitory neurotransmitter gamma-aminobutyric acid (GABA).

Indications. VPA is now established as effective over the complete range of seizure types, with particular value for the idiopathic generalized epilepsies.

Dosage. The starting dose for adults and adolescents should be 500 mg once or twice daily. Alterations thereafter can be made according to the clinical status of the patient. Divalproex sodium (a combination of valproic acid and VPA) can also be given twice daily. As the drug can take several weeks to become fully effective, frequent dose adjustments shortly after therapy is started may be unwarranted. Because VPA does not exhibit a clear-cut concentration–effect–toxicity relationship and daily variations in concentration at a given dose are wide, routine monitoring is not helpful unless closely correlated with the patient's clinical situation. A few patients need and tolerate serum concentrations up to 150 mg/liter.

Side effects. Unpleasant side effects include dose-related tremor, weight gain due to appetite stimulation, thinning or loss of hair (usually temporary) and menstrual irregularities including amenorrhea. Some young women develop polycystic ovarian syndrome associated with obesity and hirsutism. Rarely, stupor and encephalopathy associated with hyperammonemia can occur. The insidious development of parkinsonism has also been reported, although this effect reverses on VPA withdrawal. Hepatotoxicity, histologically a microvesicular steatosis similar to that found in Reye's syndrome, affects fewer than 1 in 20 000 exposed individuals. This appears to be a particular concern in children under 3 years of age receiving AED polypharmacy, some of whom will have a coexistent metabolic defect. Other sporadic problems include thrombocytopenia and pancreatitis.

An important concern in women of childbearing potential is an increased risk of major malformations in their offspring if they are exposed to VPA in the first trimester of pregnancy. Recent data from prospective pregnancy registries suggest the risk may be up to 6%, including an estimated 1–3% risk of neural tube defect. The risk appears to be higher when VPA is taken in high doses (over 1000 mg/day) or in combination with certain other AEDs, particularly LTG and CBZ. Because of its teratogenic risk, it is now recommended that women of childbearing potential should not be started on VPA without specialist neurological advice.

Pharmacokinetics and drug–drug interactions. VPA can inhibit a range of hepatic metabolic processes, including oxidation, conjugation and epoxidation reactions. Targets include other AEDs, particularly PHT, phenobarbital (PB), the active epoxide metabolite of CBZ and LTG. VPA does not, however, interfere metabolically with the hormonal components of the oral contraceptive pill.

Ethosuximide (ESM) was introduced in 1958. It works by reducing T-type calcium currents in thalamic neurons.

Indications. Since its introduction, ESM has been the drug of choice for children with absence seizures who do not also have tonic–clonic or myoclonic seizures. ESM is also effective for atypical absences, but ineffective for myoclonic, tonic–clonic and partial-onset seizures.

Dosage. In adults, dosing is initiated with 500 mg daily (250 mg/day in children less than 6 years old), with 250-mg dose increments as clinically indicated over 2–3 weeks to the maximum tolerated amount, which is typically 15–40 mg/kg given two or three times daily. Serum concentrations less than 40 mg/liter are usually ineffective.

Side effects occur in approximately 40% of patients and predominantly relate to the gastrointestinal tract (hiccups, nausea, vomiting, abdominal pain, anorexia). Headache, dizziness, drowsiness and unsteadiness may also occur. Allergic rashes are seen in up to 5% of patients. A transient leukopenia has been described.

Pharmacokinetics and drug–drug interactions. The metabolism of ESM is hepatic, protein binding is minimal and drug interactions are not a major problem.

Phenobarbital (PB), synthesized in 1912, is the oldest AED in common clinical use. It enhances the effect of GABA by prolonging chloride channel opening at the $GABA_A$ receptor, resulting in neuronal hyperpolarization.

Indications. Once widely prescribed for partial and tonic–clonic seizures, it is now regarded as second-line therapy in some countries because it so often causes sedation and behavioral problems (see Side effects, below). Nevertheless, on a global scale PB remains one of the most important AEDs because of its continuing widespread use in the developing world and in many industrialized countries. The parenteral formulation of PB is occasionally useful as adjunctive therapy in SE. PB may also be used for myoclonic seizures.

Dosage. In children, doses of 2–5 mg/kg daily are usually necessary for optimal seizure control. Resulting serum concentrations typically range from 15 to 40 mg/liter. Maintenance dosage in adults ranges from 60 to 240 mg/day. Tapering PB medication should be attempted slowly (e.g. 15 mg/month) to minimize the possibility of withdrawal seizures and other unpleasant symptoms, such as altered mood and sleep disturbance.

Side effects. As mentioned above, PB often causes sedation and behavioral problems, such as depression and agitation. In addition, it may cause hyperactivity in children and elderly patients. Recent data from the US pregnancy registry suggests an increased risk of fetal abnormalities in children born to women taking PB.

Pharmacokinetics and drug–drug interactions. PB is metabolized in the liver, and is a powerful inducer of hepatic metabolism, accelerating the clearance of many other lipid-soluble drugs. The half-life of PB is 4 days. Consequently, steady-state serum concentrations may not be reached for up to 3 weeks after a change in dose.

Primidone (PRM) is metabolized in the liver to PB and another active substance, phenylethylmalonamide. It is not fully understood how much of a role the latter plays in the overall antiepileptic effect of PRM.

Indications. PRM is effective against partial and generalized tonic–clonic seizures, but appeared to be inferior to CBZ and PHT in clinical trials, largely because of its relative poor tolerability (see below). Therefore, it is primarily used as adjunctive therapy.

Dosage. Dosing should be started with 125 mg at bedtime, increasing by 125 mg every 3–5 days as tolerated to 500–1500 mg daily in two or three divided doses. As with PB, discontinuation of PRM should be very gradual.

Side effects. PRM has a higher incidence of side effects than CBZ, PHT and PB, particularly sedation and ataxia. Decreased libido or impotence associated with PRM use has been reported.

Pharmacokinetics and drug–drug interactions. As its half-life is shorter than that of PB, concentrations of PB are usually higher than those of PRM. Like PB, PRM is a powerful enzyme inducer.

Clonazepam (CZP), like other benzodiazepines, enhances GABA-mediated inhibition.

Indications. CZP is primarily used as adjunctive treatment for generalized seizures such as absence, myoclonic and atonic seizures. It is also effective against partial and tonic–clonic seizures. Parenteral CZP can be used for SE.

Dosage. Adults should be started on 0.5–1.0 mg/day with subsequent weekly increments as necessary. In children, 0.5 mg/day is the usual starting dose. Tolerance to the anticonvulsant effect and difficulty weaning patients off CZP limit its clinical value.

Side effects are prominent, usually dose limiting, and include sedation, ataxia and behavioral changes, such as depression.

Pharmacokinetics and drug–drug interactions. Drug interactions of CZP are minimal, although its half-life in adults can be slightly reduced from 17–56 hours (as monotherapy) to 12–46 hours in the presence of an enzyme-inducing AED.

Clobazam (CLB). CLB's structure (1,5-benzodiazepine) differs slightly from those of CZP and diazepam (1,4-benzodiazepines), which may account for CLB's lower propensity to produce sedation.

Indications. CLB is a useful adjunctive drug for refractory partial and generalized seizures. CLB is not available in the USA.

Dosage. Short-term administration (e.g. 20 mg daily for 3 days) can be an effective strategy in women with premenstrual seizure exacerbations and as 'cover' for holidays or stressful events, such as weddings and surgery. A single dose of 10–30 mg can have a useful prophylactic action if taken immediately after the first event in patients who regularly suffer clusters of complex partial and secondary generalized seizures.

Not all responders will maintain a worthwhile improvement in seizure control on long-term dosing owing to the development of tolerance. Nevertheless, a substantial proportion (10–20%) of patients treated with CLB become seizure free. Intermittent use of CLB reduces the likelihood of tolerance.

Side effects. As already mentioned, CLB is less likely to cause sedation than the 1,4-benzodiazepines. Nevertheless, depression, irritability and tiredness are reported. As with barbiturates, deterioration in behavior and mood disturbance can occur, particularly in patients with learning disabilities; CLB should probably be avoided in such patients.

Pharmacokinetics and drug–drug interactions. CLB is biotransformed in the liver to a number of metabolites, including an active metabolite *N*-desmethylclobazam. Comedication with enzyme-inducing AEDs increases the metabolism of CLB, and hence the *N*-desmethylclobazam level. The clinical relevance of this interaction has not been established.

Modern antiepileptic drugs

After a hiatus of nearly 20 years, ten new AEDs (and one device – the vagus nerve stimulator [see page 89]) have received licenses for the adjunctive treatment of refractory epilepsy. Lamotrigine (LTG), gabapentin (GBP), topiramate (TPM), oxcarbazepine (OXC), tiagabine (TGB) and levetiracetam (LEV) are widely available. Zonisamide (ZNS) and pregabalin (PGB) are in the process of being marketed around the world. The progress of felbamate (FBM) has been dramatically curtailed because of the unusual development of idiosyncratic life-threatening bone-marrow and liver toxicity. The use of vigabatrin

TABLE 5.4

Pharmacological properties of new antiepileptic drugs

Drug	Primary mode(s) of action	Indications (type of seizure/syndrome)
Felbamate	Multiple	Partial onset, Lennox–Gastaut
Gabapentin	Neuronal calcium-channel binding	Partial onset
Lamotrigine	Sodium-channel blockade	Partial, generalized
Levetiracetam	Uncertain	Partial onset
Oxcarbazepine	Sodium-channel blockade	Partial, GTCS
Pregabalin	Neuronal calcium-channel binding	Partial onset
Tiagabine	GABAergic	Partial onset
Topiramate	Multiple	Partial, GTCS, myoclonic, Lennox–Gastaut
Vigabatrin	GABAergic	Partial onset
Zonisamide	Multiple	Partial, GTCS

*As monotherapy.
†Parameters for active metabolite 10-hydroxycarbamazepine.

(VGB) has also been markedly restricted because of reports of concentric visual-field defects in up to 40% of patients. The advent of these newer treatments has provided many more options in the management of refractory epilepsy.

Some of these AEDs, namely LTG, GBP, OXC and TPM, have also demonstrated efficacy as monotherapy in newly diagnosed epilepsy and have received approval for this indication in some countries. The pharmacological properties of these newer AEDs are highlighted in Table 5.4. Dosing information in adults and children is summarized in Tables 5.5 and 5.6, respectively.

Absorption (bioavailability %)	Protein binding (% bound)	Elimination half-life* (hours)	Routes of elimination
Slow (95–100)	22–36	13–23	Hepatic metabolism Renal excretion
Slow (60)	0	6–9	Not metabolized Renal excretion
Rapid (95–100)	55	22–36	Glucuronidation
Rapid (95–100)	< 10	7–8	Non-hepatic hydrolysis Renal excretion
Rapid (95–100)	40†	8–10†	Hepatic conversion to active moiety
Rapid (90–100)	0	6	Not metabolized Renal excretion
Rapid (95–100)	96	5–9	Hepatic metabolism
Slow (80)	9–17	20–24	Hepatic metabolism Renal excretion
Slow (60–80)	0	5–7	Not metabolized Renal excretion
Rapid (95–100)	40–60	50–68	Hepatic metabolism Renal excretion

GABA, gamma-aminobutyric acid; GTCS, generalized tonic–clonic seizures.

TABLE 5.5

Dosing guidelines for new antiepileptic drugs in adults

Drug	Starting dose (mg/day)	Commonest dose (mg/day)	Maintenance range (mg/day)	Dosing interval
Felbamate	1200	2400	1800–4800	tds
Gabapentin	300–400	2400	1200–4800	tds
Lamotrigine	12.5–25*	200–400	100–800	od–bd
Levetiracetam	1000	2000–3000	1000–4000	bd
Oxcarbazepine	150–600	900–1800	900–2700	bd–tds
Pregabalin	150	300	150–600	bd–tds
Tiagabine	4–10	40	20–60	bd–qds
Topiramate	25–50	200–400	100–1000	bd
Vigabatrin	500–1000	3000	2000–4000	od–bd
Zonisamide	100	400	400–600	od–bd

*12.5 mg with sodium valproate (every other day in the USA); 25 mg as monotherapy. Also see Table 5.7 for schedules recommended for add-on or monotherapy use.
od, once daily; bd, twice daily; tds, three times a day; qds, four times a day.

Lamotrigine (LTG) selectively blocks the slow inactivated state of the sodium channel, thereby preventing the release of excitatory amino-acid neurotransmitters, particularly glutamate and aspartate. This mode of action does not explain its antiabsence and antimyoclonic properties.

Indications. LTG appears to be effective across the complete range of seizure types, including partial seizures, the idiopathic generalized epilepsies and Lennox–Gastaut syndrome. It is licensed widely as add-on treatment for adults with refractory epilepsy. Its use in children and as monotherapy in newly diagnosed epilepsy has been approved in a growing number of countries. Good results have been reported in patients with learning disabilities, who often have multiple seizure types. LTG's ability to reduce interictal spiking may explain the improved alertness reported by some people taking the drug. Its efficacy may be enhanced when combined with VPA, although this combination is

TABLE 5.6

Dosing guidelines for new antiepileptic drugs in children

Drug	Starting dose (mg/kg/day)	Maintenance dose (mg/kg/day)	Dosing interval
Felbamate	15	30–45	tds–qds
Gabapentin*	20	20–40	tds
Lamotrigine			
– monotherapy	0.5	2–8	od–bd
– with valproate	0.15	1–5	od–bd
Levetiracetam	10	20–60	bd
Oxcarbazepine	5	10–50	bd–tds
Pregabalin*†	–	–	–
Tiagabine*†	–	–	–
Topiramate	0.5–1 (od)	5–9	bd
Vigabatrin	40	50–150	od–bd
Zonisamide	2–4	4–8	bd

*Not approved for use in pediatric population.
†Not yet recommended for children under 12 years of age.
od, once daily; bd, twice daily; tds, three times a day; qds, four times a day.

associated with higher rates of rash, tremor and teratogenesis. Recent reports suggest that LTG may exacerbate myoclonic seizures in some patients, particularly those with severe myoclonic epilepsy.

Dosage. LTG can be administered once daily as monotherapy or with VPA, or twice daily in patients taking enzyme-inducing AEDs. A low starting dose with a slow titration schedule will reduce the risk of rash. This depends on concomitant medication (Table 5.7). Some patients respond to and tolerate doses exceeding 600 mg daily as monotherapy, or above 800 mg daily in combination with an enzyme-inducing AED. An equivalent high dose in VPA-treated patients would be 150–200 mg daily because of the extent of metabolic inhibition. With the above exceptions, routine concentration monitoring is not required, as no useful relationship has been established between LTG concentrations and its anticonvulsant efficacy or the emergence of side effects.

TABLE 5.7

Lamotrigine dosing and titration schedules

As add-on therapy	Concomitant antiepileptic drugs	
Adults		
	Valproate	Others
Weeks 1 and 2	12.5 mg daily*	50 mg daily
Weeks 3 and 4	25 mg daily†	50 mg twice daily
Maintenance	50–100 mg‡ twice daily	100–200 mg‡ twice daily
Children		
	Valproate	Others
Weeks 1 and 2	0.15 mg/kg	0.6 mg/kg
Weeks 3 and 4	0.3 mg/kg	1.2 mg/kg
Increments	0.3 mg/kg	1.2 mg/kg
Maintenance	1–5 mg/kg‡	5–15 mg/kg‡
As monotherapy	**Adults**	**Children**
Weeks 1 and 2	25 mg daily	0.5 mg/kg
Weeks 3 and 4	25 mg twice daily	1 mg/kg
Maintenance	50–100 mg‡ twice daily	2–8 mg/kg‡

*12.5 mg every other day is more common in the USA.
†12.5 mg daily is more common in the USA.
‡Higher doses can be tried if seizures persist and patient's tolerance is good.

Side effects include headache, nausea, insomnia, vomiting, dizziness, diplopia, ataxia and tremor. The drug seldom causes sedation. Rash complicates initial management in around 3% of patients taking LTG as monotherapy, and in 8% of those already established on VPA. It is usually maculopapular and, in mild cases, may subside spontaneously without drug withdrawal. In a few patients, however, there is an accompanying systemic illness with malaise, fever, arthralgia, myalgia, lymphadenopathy and eosinophilia. Cases of bullous erythema multiforme, Stevens–Johnson syndrome and toxic epidermal necrolysis have also been reported. The risk of a severe skin reaction may be as high as 1 in 1000 adults and 1 in 100 children. Gradual introduction of LTG lessens the likelihood of rash, so the prescribing guidelines should be religiously adhered to. Preliminary results from large-scale pregnancy registries suggest only a small risk of major fetal malformation associated with LTG monotherapy, similar to that associated with CBZ (approximately 2.5%); however, this risk may be considerably higher (up to 11%) when the drug is given with VPA.

Pharmacokinetics and drug–drug interactions. LTG does not influence the metabolism of lipid-soluble drugs, including other AEDs, warfarin and the oral contraceptive pill. As monotherapy, the half-life approximates 24 hours. When LTG is given to patients already being treated with the enzyme-inducing agents CBZ, PHT or PB, the half-life falls to about 15 hours. VPA inhibits LTG's glucuronidation, prolonging its half-life to around 60 hours. Withdrawal of enzyme-inducing AEDs, therefore, causes a rise in the circulating concentrations of LTG, while discontinuing VPA produces a fall.

Serum concentrations of LTG fall dramatically during pregnancy and also in patients starting an estrogen-containing oral contraceptive. In these circumstances, concentration monitoring may be helpful in guiding LTG dose adjustment.

A pharmacodynamic interaction resulting in symptoms of neurotoxicity (headache, dizziness, nausea, diplopia, ataxia) is a common consequence when LTG is introduced in patients established on high-dose CBZ. This effect can be reduced by staggering doses of CBZ and LTG by 2–3 hours instead of simultaneous administration. A pharmacodynamic interaction has also been proposed as the explanation for the marked tremor seen in some patients taking VPA and LTG in combination.

Gabapentin (GBP) was formed by adding a cyclohexyl group to GABA, which allowed it to cross the blood–brain barrier. Despite its structure, GBP does not bind to GABA receptors in the CNS. It appears to work by binding to the $\alpha 2$-δ subunit of the neuronal voltage-gated calcium channels, inhibiting calcium flow and neurotransmitter release from presynaptic neurons.

Indications. GBP is approved as adjunctive therapy for partial seizures with or without secondary generalization in patients 12 years of age or older. It has also been licensed as monotherapy for these types of seizures in some countries. It may exacerbate myoclonic jerks and generalized absences. In addition, GBP is useful for the treatment of neuropathic pain.

Dosage. Dosing should be initiated at 300 mg or 400 mg a day and increased by 300-mg or 400-mg increments every 1–3 days to the maximum tolerated dose using a thrice-daily regimen. The recommended dose range is 1200–2400 mg daily (900–1800 mg daily in the USA). However, many patients with refractory epilepsy will need higher amounts (up to 4800 mg daily) for optimal seizure control.

Side effects with GBP are generally mild and transient. Drowsiness, ataxia, dizziness and nystagmus are the most common. Weight gain occurs in up to 5% of patients, particularly at higher doses. Flatulence, diarrhea and myoclonic jerks have also been reported. No idiosyncratic reactions or effects on bone marrow or hepatic function have been described.

Pharmacokinetics and drug–drug interactions. GBP is not metabolized, and does not induce or inhibit hepatic enzymes. Drug interactions, therefore, are not an issue with this agent. Its half-life is 6–9 hours. GBP is eliminated unchanged by the kidneys, so patients with renal insufficiency need lower doses and less frequent dosing. A useful serum concentration range has not been established.

Vigabatrin (VGB). VGB's antiepileptic effect is mediated by suicidal inhibition of GABA transaminase, the enzyme responsible for the metabolic degradation of GABA (Figure 5.4).

Indications. VGB is an effective add-on drug for patients with partial seizures with or without secondary generalization. It can worsen myoclonic jerks and generalized absences.

Unfortunately, its usefulness has been severely limited by the development of visual-field constriction in up to 40% of patients. This problem was first noted 8 years after the initial launch of the drug. As a result, VGB is only recommended as adjunctive therapy for partial seizures when there is no other alternative. However, VGB

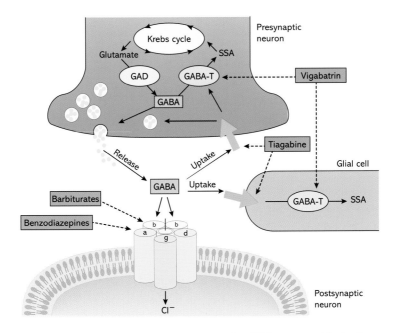

Figure 5.4 Effects of vigabatrin and tiagabine at the GABA$_A$ receptor. Vigabatrin inhibits GABA-T, which degrades GABA, and tiagabine blocks presynaptic neuronal and glial uptake of synaptically released GABA. GABA, gamma-aminobutyric acid; GABA-T, GABA transaminase; GAD, glutamic acid decarboxylase; SSA, succinic semi-aldehyde. With permission from Leach JP and Brodie MJ. Tiagabine. © *Lancet* 1998;351:204.

is still regarded by many pediatric neurologists as the treatment of choice for infantile spasms; more than 50% of children have been reported as spasm free after 1 week of treatment. Children with tuberous sclerosis often have a particularly favorable response.

Dosage. VGB is usually added to existing AED therapy, initially in a dose of 500 mg once or twice daily to allow tolerance to any sedation. If the patient complains of agitation or a thought disorder, the drug should be withdrawn immediately. Further increments of 500 mg or 1000 mg daily will depend on the clinical status of the patient. Seizures in most patients will respond to 2000–3000 mg daily. Few show further improvement at higher doses. Children should start treatment at 40 mg/kg daily, increased according to response up to

80–100 mg/kg daily. Infants with spasms may need as much as 150 mg/kg daily. When being discontinued, VGB should be tapered slowly, as abrupt cessation can produce a marked increase in seizures and can precipitate psychosis. Monitoring of VGB concentrations is unnecessary as the drug does not exhibit a useful concentration–effect–toxicity relationship.

Side effects. Tiredness, dizziness, headache and weight gain are the most frequent adverse effects with VGB. Some patients report a change in mood, commonly agitation, ill temper, disturbed behavior or depression. Paranoid and psychotic symptoms can develop. It can cause hyperkinesia and agitation in children. No idiosyncratic reactions have been reported with VGB. For patients in whom the benefit of VGB treatment is judged to outweigh the risk of visual-field constriction (as discussed above), formal visual-field monitoring should be performed regularly. There is no evidence that VGB is a human teratogen.

Pharmacokinetics and drug–drug interactions. VGB does not interfere with hepatic metabolic enzymes, but produces a small reduction in PHT levels of around 20% by an unknown mechanism.

Topiramate (TPM) is a sulfamate-substituted monosaccharide that has multiple pharmacological actions involving blockade of sodium channels and high-voltage-activated calcium channels, attenuation of kainate-induced responses and enhancement of GABAergic neurotransmission. It also inhibits carbonic anhydrase, an effect that contributes to its side-effect profile.

Indications. TPM has proven efficacy against partial and tonic–clonic seizures. It also seems effective in myoclonic epilepsies, including some of the more severe syndromes of childhood. A useful effect on generalized absences has yet to be shown. However, it can provide benefit to patients with Lennox–Gastaut syndrome and possibly also infantile spasms. TPM has similar effectiveness to CBZ or VPA as monotherapy for partial and generalized seizures, and has received a monotherapy indication for newly diagnosed epilepsy in some countries. In addition to its indication for the treatment of epilepsy, TPM is also approved for migraine prophylaxis.

Dosage. Patients respond to TPM in doses ranging from 50–1000 mg daily. It is administered in two divided doses and should be introduced slowly. An initial dose of 25–50 mg daily can be increased by 25–50 mg every 1–2 weeks until a maximally effective and/or tolerated dose is achieved. The optimum amount for most patients with refractory epilepsy appears to be 200–400 mg twice daily. Higher doses (400–800 mg daily) may be required in patients taking PHT or CBZ, with lower amounts (100–200 mg) often being successful in those taking non-enzyme-inducing AEDs. Some patients respond to doses as low as 50–100 mg daily, particularly if TPM is combined with LTG. Concentration monitoring of TPM is not required. However, measurement of PHT levels may be necessary in patients who develop symptoms suggestive of toxicity. Women taking an oral contraceptive should use a formulation containing at least 50 µg of ethinylestradiol if the daily dose of TPM exceeds 200 mg.

Side effects related to the CNS include ataxia, poor concentration, confusion, dysphasia, dizziness, fatigue, paresthesia, somnolence, word-finding difficulties and cognitive slowing. The risk of neurocognitive side effects can be minimized by titrating up the dose slowly. Anorexia and weight loss are common accompaniments of TPM therapy. It increases the risk of nephrolithiasis tenfold and, therefore, should be avoided in patients with a history of kidney stones and in those taking calcium supplements or high-dose vitamin C. In preclinical studies involving mice, rats and rabbits, TPM was found to be teratogenic at high doses. It is therefore not advised for use during pregnancy, unless the benefits of treatment are felt to outweigh the potential risk to the fetus.

Pharmacokinetics and drug–drug interactions. TPM inhibits the metabolism of PHT in about 10% of patients. When used in doses over 200 mg/day, it can accelerate the breakdown of the estrogenic component of the oral contraceptive pill. PHT and CBZ induce TPM degradation, reducing its concentration by 40% or more.

Tiagabine (TGB) selectively inhibits the neuronal and glial reuptake of GABA, and thereby enhances GABA-mediated inhibition (see Figure 5.4).

Indications. TGB is licensed throughout the EU, and has been approved for use in the USA as add-on therapy in refractory partial epilepsy.

Dosage. It is available as 5-mg, 10-mg and 15-mg tablets, except in the USA, Canada and Mexico where 2-mg, 4-mg, 12-mg, 16-mg and 20-mg tablets of TGB are produced. Studies suggest a minimal effective dose of around 20–30 mg/day as add-on therapy in partial epilepsy. The dose range most extensively studied has been 32–56 mg/day, but some patients have demonstrated benefit with up to 80 mg daily. Dosing is likely to be substantially lower when the drug is used as monotherapy. Treatment in adults is started with 4–5 mg once or twice daily, followed by weekly increments of 4–5 mg. A change to three-times-daily dosing is recommended when 30 mg or more of the drug is prescribed daily. TGB should be taken with food to avoid rapid rises in plasma concentration. Routine plasma level monitoring is not required.

Side effects include dizziness, asthenia (fatigue or muscle weakness), nervousness, tremor, impaired concentration, lethargy and depression. Weakness due to transient loss of tone can occur at high doses. The commonest reasons for discontinuation of therapy are confusion, somnolence, ataxia and dizziness. In clinical trials, TGB-treated patients experienced similar rates of occurrence for rash and psychosis as those taking placebo. The safety of TGB in pregnancy is unknown, but it is not teratogenic in animals at therapeutic doses. Absence stupor has been reported as a rare side effect.

Pharmacokinetics and drug–drug interactions. TGB is rapidly and completely absorbed. Food reduces the rate, but not the extent, of absorption. TGB is extensively metabolized by hepatic oxidization via the cytochrome P450 (CYP450) isoenzyme CYP3A. Because TGB does not induce or inhibit liver enzymes, concentrations of CBZ, PHT, theophylline, warfarin and digoxin are unaffected. VPA levels may drop slightly by an unknown mechanism. TGB's half-life is 5–9 hours, falling to 2–4 hours when the drug is coadministered with hepatic enzyme-inducing AEDs, such as CBZ and PHT. TGB undergoes linear pharmacokinetics that do not vary greatly in the elderly. Lower doses are required in patients with substantial hepatic, but not renal, impairment.

Oxcarbazepine (OXC), the 10-keto analog of CBZ, is licensed worldwide. It is functionally a prodrug, being rapidly reduced in the liver to the active metabolite 10,11-dihydro-10-hydroxycarbamazepine. Principally, it prevents burst firing of neurons by blocking sodium channels, but it also modulates calcium and potassium currents.

Indications. OXC has a similar spectrum of efficacy to CBZ against partial and tonic–clonic seizures. It tends to be better tolerated than CBZ with fewer neurotoxic side effects.

Dosage. The recommended starting dose for OXC in adults is 150–600 mg daily in two doses. The dose can be titrated upwards as clinically indicated to 3000–4000 mg daily. A starting dose of 5 mg/kg daily in children over 3 years of age can be prescribed initially, increasing gradually to a maintenance amount of about 30 mg/kg daily.

Patients already on CBZ may be switched immediately to OXC using a dosage ratio of 1.5 (OXC) to 1 (CBZ). Particular care in immediate switching needs to be taken when the daily CBZ dose exceeds 1200 mg. Plasma concentrations of the clinically active metabolite of OXC increase linearly with dose. No studies, however, have attempted to relate elevated plasma levels with efficacy or toxicity.

Side effects most often involve the CNS and include drowsiness, dizziness, headache, diplopia, nausea, vomiting and ataxia. Rash occurs less frequently with OXC than with CBZ, but like CBZ, OXC has been implicated in rare cases of Stevens–Johnson syndrome and toxic epidermal necrolysis. OXC does not appear to produce blood dyscrasias or hepatotoxicity. Hyponatremia, which is not clearly due to an antidiuretic hormone-like effect, is somewhat more common with OXC than with CBZ, although affected patients are rarely symptomatic. There is no evidence that OXC is a human teratogen, although high doses produce malformations in rodents.

Pharmacokinetics and drug–drug interactions. OXC has no effect on its own metabolism, but it induces a single isoform of CYP450, resulting in accelerated clearance of the hormonal components of the oral contraceptive pill.

Felbamate (FBM) potentiates GABA activity and blocks voltage-dependent sodium channels as well as the ionic channel at the N-methyl-D-aspartate excitatory amino-acid receptor.

Indications. FBM has demonstrated effectiveness both as monotherapy and add-on therapy for partial-onset seizures with or without secondary generalization in patients 14 years of age or older. It also has important efficacy as adjunctive therapy in the treatment of partial and generalized seizures (including atonic seizures) associated with the Lennox–Gastaut syndrome in children.

Dosage. Dosing should be initiated slowly and titrated over several weeks to minimize side effects. Doses of 1800–4800 mg daily in adults and 15–45 mg/kg daily in children are usually necessary for optimal seizure control. Routine monitoring of liver and bone marrow function is recommended, but will not fully predict potentially fatal toxicity.

Side effects include insomnia, headache, nausea, anorexia, somnolence, vomiting, weight loss and dizziness. Clinical experience with FBM subsequent to its approval by the US Food and Drug Administration showed a notable incidence of aplastic anemia and hepatotoxicity. As a result, the use of FBM is now largely restricted to patients with Lennox–Gastaut syndrome for whom the benefits of treatment outweigh the risks.

Pharmacokinetics and drug–drug interactions. In total, 25% of FBM is bound to plasma protein and approximately 50% is metabolized by the hepatic CYP450 system. Its half-life ranges from 15–24 hours. FBM increases serum concentrations of PHT, VPA and CBZ epoxide. Thus, dose adjustment of concomitant AEDs is usually necessary when FBM is introduced.

Levetiracetam (LEV) is an enantiomer of the ethyl analog of piracetam. It differs from other AEDs in its preclinical profile; unlike other AEDs, it does not act by GABA facilitation, inhibition of sodium channels or modulation of calcium currents. Although several modes of action have been suggested – such as suppression of negative allosteric modulators on neuronal GABA- and glycine-gated currents, reduction of voltage-operated potassium currents and binding to synaptic vesicle protein – LEV's exact mechanism of action remains uncertain.

Indications. LEV is approved for use in adults and in children of 4 years of age and older. It has proven efficacy for treatment-resistant partial seizures, and there is increasing evidence of efficacy in a variety of generalized seizure types, including myoclonic jerks and absences.

Dosage. In controlled studies, patients with partial seizures responded to 1000–3000 mg daily. Daily doses of up to 4000 mg appear to be well tolerated. Treatment can be initiated at 250–500 mg twice daily and titrated at 1000-mg increments every 2 weeks as tolerated and needed for seizure control. Urinary excretion of unchanged drug accounts for approximately 60% of an administered dose, so patients with moderate-to-severe renal impairment may need lower amounts at longer intervals.

Side effects. LEV is generally well tolerated. The most common side effect is sleepiness or somnolence. Some patients complain of headache, anorexia and nervousness. Behavioral problems such as agitation, aggression, hostility, psychosis, anxiety and depression have been reported in up to 7% of patients, particularly those with a prior history of psychiatric illness. The risk of behavioral side effects can be reduced by adopting a slower titration schedule. To date, no idiosyncratic reactions have been reported.

Pharmacokinetics and drug–drug interactions. LEV is less than 10% protein bound. The major metabolic pathway is hydrolysis of the acetamide group to the inactive carboxylic derivative. Because its metabolism is independent of the hepatic CYP450 system, there are no pharmacokinetic interactions with other drugs, including oral contraceptives. Steady state is achieved after 2 days of twice-daily dosing. Children aged 6–12 years clear LEV faster than adults. In young adults, the half-life is 7–8 hours, compared with 10–11 hours in the healthy elderly, who have age-related diminished renal function.

Zonisamide (ZNS) is a sulfonamide derivative, chemically and structurally unrelated to other AEDs. It blocks voltage-dependent sodium and T-type calcium channels, and actively inhibits the release of excitatory neurotransmitters. Although probably not a major contributor to ZNS's pharmacological effect, its weak inhibition of carbonic anhydrase activity may contribute to its side-effect profile.

Indications. ZNS has proven efficacy for treatment-resistant partial seizures. Evidence also suggests efficacy for infantile spasms and a variety of generalized seizure types, including tonic–clonic, tonic, atonic and atypical absence seizures. Anecdotal reports suggest that ZNS may have important benefits against myoclonic seizures, particularly in patients with progressive myoclonic epilepsy.

Dosage. The recommended initial dose for ZNS is 100 mg daily for adult patients, and 2 mg/kg/day for children in two divided doses. Because steady state is reached slowly, the dose should be increased at 2-week intervals to a target maintenance amount of 400–600 mg/day in adults and 4–8 mg/kg/day in children.

Side effects include anorexia, dizziness, ataxia, fatigue, somnolence, confusion and poor concentration. Gastrointestinal problems and loss of or decrease in spontaneity have been described. Around 2% of treated patients develop renal stones that may resolve spontaneously.

Pharmacokinetics and drug–drug interactions. Approximately 40% of ZNS is protein bound in serum; it is unaffected by tightly protein-bound drugs, and it has no effect on hepatic metabolism. ZNS has a high affinity for erythrocytes, and this binding is saturable; the relationship between the dose and whole-blood ZNS concentration is therefore non-linear at high doses. The plasma half-life of ZNS is 50–68 hours, so steady state is achieved in about 15 days. Children require higher daily doses than adults to achieve comparable serum concentrations because of faster clearance. Patients with renal dysfunction have lower rates of clearance. Enzyme-inducing AEDs, such as PHT, CBZ and PB, decrease the half-life of ZNS by approximately 50%.

Pregabalin (PGB) is the latest AED to receive approval. It has an amino acid configuration and is structurally related to GABA. Like GBP, it binds with high affinity to the α2-δ subunit of neuronal voltage-gated calcium channels. However, it is six to eight times more potent than GBP.

Indications. PGB is licensed as adjunctive treatment for partial seizures with or without secondary generalization. It has also shown benefit for neuropathic pain and generalized anxiety disorder.

Key points – antiepileptic drugs

- Ten new antiepileptic drugs (AEDs) have been approved for the treatment of epilepsy since the late 1980s.
- AEDs differ substantially in their mechanisms of action, spectra of activity, and pharmacokinetic and side-effect profiles.
- The wider choice of AEDs now available permits the drug to be matched to the individual patient's circumstances.

Dosage. The recommended starting dose is 150 mg daily, usually given in divided doses without titration. The maximum dose used in regulatory trials was 600 mg daily, which can be prescribed as 300 mg twice daily or 200 mg three times daily.

Side effects include dizziness, somnolence, asthenia, headache and ataxia. Patients may experience weight gain, particularly at high doses. Peripheral edema has also been noted. Serious adverse events, including rash and other idiosyncratic reactions, have not been reported with this new AED.

Pharmacokinetics and drug–drug interactions. PGB's absorption is rapid, linear and almost complete. The short elimination half-life of 6–8 hours led to the use of twice- and thrice-daily dosing in clinical trials. PGB is excreted unchanged by the kidney and displays no pharmacokinetic interactions with any other drug, including all AEDs. Dosage adjustment is necessary in patients with substantial renal failure and in those maintained on hemodialysis.

Key references

Brodie MJ. Pregabalin as adjunctive therapy for partial seizures. *Epilepsia* 2004;45(suppl 6):19–27.

Brodie MJ, Dichter MA. Antiepileptic drugs. *N Engl J Med* 1996;334:168–75.

Brodie MJ, Dichter MA. Established antiepileptic drugs. *Seizure* 1997;6: 159–74.

Dichter MA, Brodie MJ. New antiepileptic drugs. *N Engl J Med* 1996;334:1583–90.

French JA, Kanner AM, Bautista J et al. Efficacy and tolerability of the new antiepileptic drugs I: treatment of new onset epilepsy. Report of the Therapeutics and Technology Assessment Subcommittee and Quality Standards Subcommittee of the American Academy of Neurology and the American Epilepsy Society. *Neurology* 2004;62:1252–60.

French JA, Kanner AM, Bautista J et al. Efficacy and tolerability of the new antiepileptic drugs II: treatment of refractory epilepsy. Report of the Therapeutics and Technology Assessment Committee and Quality Standards Subcommittee of the American Academy of Neurology and the American Epilepsy Society. *Neurology* 2004;62:1261–73.

Kwan P, Brodie MJ. Phenobarbital for the treatment of epilepsy in the 21st century: a critical review. *Epilepsia* 2004;45:1141–9.

Marson AG, Hutton JL, Leach JP et al. Levetiracetam, oxcarbazepine, remacemide and zonisamide for drug resistant localization-related epilepsy: a systematic review. *Epilepsy Res* 2001;46:259–70.

Marson AG, Kadir ZA, Hutton JL, Chadwick DW. The new antiepileptic drugs: a systematic review of their efficacy and tolerability. *Epilepsia* 1997;38:859–80.

National Institute for Clinical Excellence. TA076 – Newer drugs for epilepsy in adults, full guidance. Technology Appraisal 76. London: NICE, March 2004. www.nice.org.uk/TA076guidance

Pellock JM. Managing pediatric epilepsy syndromes with new antiepileptic drugs. *Pediatrics* 1999;104:1106–16.

Schmidt D, Elger CE. What is the evidence that oxcarbazepine and carbamazepine are distinctly different antiepileptic drugs? *Epilepsy Behav* 2004;5:627–35.

Epilepsy surgery

Epilepsy surgery should be considered for patients with medically refractory seizures, because of the increased mortality and progressive cognitive and psychosocial morbidity associated with uncontrolled seizures over many years. Although the precise definition of 'medical intractability' is still controversial, there is emerging consensus that the failure of two monotherapy regimens using well-tolerated first-line antiepileptic drugs (AEDs), or one attempt at monotherapy and one combination regimen, should prompt referral to a specialty epilepsy center that offers surgery. In some situations, such as catastrophic epilepsy in children, patients should be referred urgently because of the risk of severe developmental disability. A case-by-case assessment is needed. In addition to results of diagnostic tests, the patient's and the family's perception of epilepsy severity despite optimal pharmacotherapy and their expectations for the future are key determinants in the decision to operate.

Types of procedure. The type of surgical procedure performed depends on the indication (Table 6.1). The most common procedure is anterior temporal lobectomy for hippocampal or mesial temporal sclerosis. In well-selected cases, 70–80% of patients can become seizure free, with a surgical mortality close to 0% and less than 5% significant morbidity (e.g. hemiparesis, hemianopia).

Some patients may be suitable candidates for a more limited resection known as amygdalohippocampectomy in which the epileptogenic hippocampus and amygdala are removed, while sparing the temporal neocortex.

Other curative procedures include lesionectomy to resect discrete structural lesions, such as glial tumors and vascular malformations. In a palliative procedure (e.g. hemispherectomy, corpus callosotomy, multiple subpial transection), the focus of the seizure is not resected. Instead, the aim of the operation is to disrupt the pathways important

TABLE 6.1

Types of epilepsy surgery and their indications

Procedure	Indication
Anterior temporal lobectomy	Mesial temporal sclerosis
Focal resection	Partial-onset seizures arising from resectable cortex
Corpus callosotomy	Tonic, atonic or tonic–clonic seizures, with falling and injury; large non-resectable lesions; secondary bilateral synchrony
Hemispherectomy	Rasmussen's syndrome or other unilateral hemisphere pathology in association with functionally impaired contralateral hand
Subpial transections	Partial-onset seizures arising from unresectable cortex

for the spread of epileptiform discharges in order to reduce the frequency and severity of the seizures. Corpus callosotomy is a treatment option for patients with severe generalized epilepsy, particularly atonic seizures with frequent falls and subsequent injuries. Multiple subpial transection is performed when the epileptogenic lesion cannot be removed due to its close proximity to the eloquent cortex, while hemispherectomy is a more drastic procedure in which an extensively diseased and epileptogenic cerebral hemisphere is removed, or left in place but is functionally disconnected.

Presurgical evaluation. There is no universally agreed protocol to identify potential surgical candidates. Presurgical evaluation aims to establish the presence of drug resistance, to delineate the epileptogenic zone to be resected and to demonstrate that its removal will not cause additional unacceptable neurological or cognitive deficits. In practice, the evaluation involves a number of processes.

- A thorough review of the patient's seizure history and AED trials is undertaken.
- Sophisticated video-electroencephalogram (EEG) monitoring localizes the onset of typical seizures.

- High-quality magnetic resonance imaging (MRI) with dedicated 'epilepsy surgery protocol' increases diagnostic accuracy.
- Functional imaging such as single photon emission computed tomography or positron emission tomography, when necessary, delineates a focal structural and/or functional lesion.
- Neuropsychological testing, including intracarotid injection of amobarbital or functional MRI, defines the laterality of language and memory functions.

Lobar excision may be carried out with a high probability of improvement when:

- EEG monitoring shows that seizure onset is consistently and repeatedly from the same portion of one frontal or temporal lobe
- other investigations are consistent with this localization
- the identified lobe can be removed safely without permanent cognitive, sensory or motor deficit.

If scalp EEG data do not clearly identify the seizure focus, or if the neuroimaging and/or neuropsychological testing results are inconsistent with the ictal results, 'invasive' electrodes may be inserted into the brain for further seizure recording (Figures 6.1–6.3). When monitoring shows that seizures arise from different sides of the brain on separate

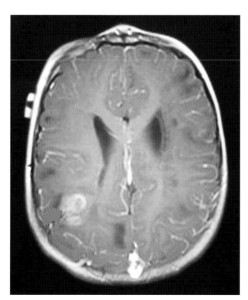

Figure 6.1 MRI scan of a patient with refractory epilepsy showing a heterogeneous lesion in the right parietal lobe (arrow).

occasions, or are consistent with generalized seizures, lobectomy is not likely to be of help. Advances in neuroimaging techniques have greatly reduced the need for invasive intracranial EEG recording.

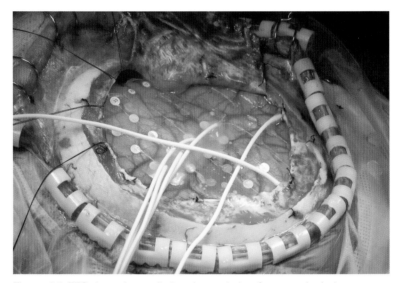

Figure 6.2 EEG electrodes applied to the cortical surface over the lesion intraoperatively to map out the area to be resected.

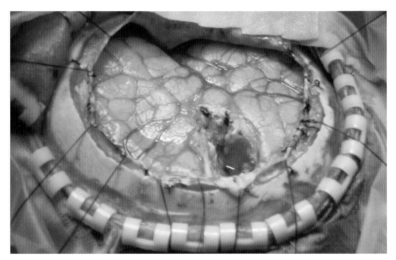

Figure 6.3 Patient in Figure 6.2 immediately after focal resection of the cortical lesion.

Vagus nerve stimulation

The introduction of vagus nerve stimulation (VNS) has provided a new, non-pharmacological approach to epilepsy treatment. Over 20 000 patients worldwide have had the VNS Therapy® system implanted. It comprises an implantable, multiprogrammable pulse generator that delivers electrical current to the vagus nerve with the aim of reducing the frequency and/or severity of epileptic seizures. VNS is approved in the USA, Canada and the EU for use as adjunctive therapy for adults and adolescents over 12 years of age whose partial-onset seizures are refractory to antiepileptic medication. Some patients with generalized seizures will also respond to VNS.

The system (Figure 6.4) consists of:
- a programmable signal generator that is implanted in the patient's left upper chest
- a bipolar lead that connects the generator to the left vagus nerve in the neck
- a programming wand that uses radio-frequency signals to communicate non-invasively with the generator
- a hand-held magnet used by the patient or carer to turn the stimulator on or off.

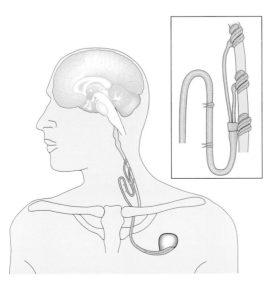

Figure 6.4 Vagus nerve stimulation (VNS) system in which the VNS pulse generator is linked by electrodes to the left vagus nerve in the neck. The enlarged section of the diagram shows how the ends of the flexible silicone leads are wound around the nerve.

89

VNS's mechanism of action is unknown. It has no effect on hepatic metabolic processes, serum concentrations of AEDs or laboratory values. It does not have a deleterious effect on vagally mediated physiological processes (as measured by Holter monitoring), pulmonary function tests or serum gastrin levels.

Implantation and setup. The implantation procedure lasts approximately 1 hour and is typically carried out under general anesthesia to minimize any possible seizure interference during surgery. Within the first 2 weeks after surgery, the output current is increased by the physician and adjusted to patient tolerance.

A typical regimen consists of a 30-Hz signal frequency with a 500-microsecond pulse width for 30 seconds of 'on time' and 5 minutes of 'off time'.

Once programmed, the generator will deliver intermittent stimulation at the desired settings until any additional instructions are received or until the battery life is expended, typically after 8–10 years of operation with the latest model. In addition, the patient or a companion may activate the generator by placing the magnet over it for several seconds; in some patients, this may interrupt a seizure or reduce its severity if applied at the onset.

Efficacy and tolerability. A number of severely affected patients treated with VNS have had clinically important seizure reductions of over 50%, and a few have become seizure free. Patients do not appear to become tolerant to the therapeutic effect induced by VNS.

Side effects are transient and include incisional pain, coughing, voice alteration, chest discomfort and nausea. Adverse effects related to stimulation are usually mild, and almost always resolve with adjustment in the settings. These include hoarseness, throat pain, coughing, dyspnea and paresthesia.

There have been no reported cognitive, sedative, visual, affective, behavioral or coordination side effects; hence, the typical central nervous system problems associated with AEDs are conspicuously absent with VNS therapy.

Ketogenic diet

The ketogenic diet is a restrictive high-fat, low-protein and very low-carbohydrate diet mostly given to children (aged 5–10 years) with medically intractable epilepsy. There is much less experience to guide its use in younger children, adolescents or adults. The diet mimics the biochemical changes associated with starvation, which creates ketosis. Its exact mechanism of seizure suppression remains unclear.

The diet was first developed in the 1920s but fell out of favor when the choice of AEDs on the market increased. However, interest in the diet has resurfaced since the early 1990s as it can be very effective in patients who have failed numerous drug trials, and it does not have the cumulative sedating effects of multiple AEDs.

Initiation and administration. The ratio of fat to carbohydrate and protein ranges from 2:1 to 4:1 (Table 6.2). Meals must be carefully chosen, with the quantities of foods strictly measured, making eating outside the home in schools or in restaurants difficult. Patients who require tube feeding can be provided with a liquid formula prepared from commercially available dietary powders. Patients are usually

TABLE 6.2

A typical day's meal for a child on a ketogenic diet*

Breakfast	Lunch	Dinner
60 g 36% heavy cream	60 g 36% heavy cream	60 g 36% heavy cream
20 g fruit	35 g vegetables	24 g vegetables
39 g eggs	19 g white tuna fish	31 g beef hotdog
22 g butter	24 g butter or margarine	14 g butter or margarine
		40 g sugar-free gelatin

*Information is based on a 5-year-old child of 18 kg bodyweight given a fat to carbohydrate and protein ratio of 4:1.
Reprinted with permission from Ballaban-Gil K. The ketogenic diet. In: Devinsky O, Westbrook LE, eds. *Epilepsy and Developmental Disabilities*. Massachusetts: Butterworth-Heinemann, 2002.

admitted for several days when the diet is initiated to monitor for any early complications such as hypoglycemia, and to educate the patient and family on how to administer the diet. Close collaboration between the patient and family, managing pediatrician and specially trained dietician is essential for successful implementation of the diet.

Efficacy and tolerability. A randomized controlled trial of the ketogenic diet has not been published, but a number of retrospective and prospective observational studies have documented more than 50% seizure reduction after 1 year on the diet in approximately 50% of children with intractable epilepsy. The diet seems to be effective in all seizure types. The major problem is adherence to the restrictive dietary regimen.

Dehydration, diarrhea and hypoglycemia may occur at the start of the diet. Common long-term side effects include weight loss or lack of weight gain, constipation and acidosis. Hyperlipidemia and renal stones are less common (6%). Rare cases of dilated cardiomyopathy, prolonged QT interval and hemorrhagic pancreatitis have been reported, but their causal relationship with the diet has not been established.

Alternative medicine

Herbal formulas have a centuries-old tradition in much of the world. Over-the-counter herbal and dietary supplements are increasingly popular with people in industrialized countries, especially patients with chronic illnesses such as epilepsy. In Japan, herbal medicines, called *kampo*, are available by prescription from physicians.

Surveys conducted in the USA and UK suggest that up to one-third of patients with epilepsy take herbs and/or dietary supplements, and that the majority of these patients do not discuss their use with their physicians. Most patients do not take the alternative medicines for seizure control, but for general maintenance of health or to control other symptoms – for example, valerian for difficulty sleeping, St John's wort for depression and *Ginkgo biloba* for memory disturbance. Thus, the particular products taken by a patient may be a clue to that patient's side effects from AEDs or comorbid disorders.

Clinicians should take a thorough history regarding herbs and dietary supplements, and consult reliable databases for information on safety as well as possible effects on seizure frequency and AED serum concentrations. Certain herbs, such as St John's wort, can affect hepatic metabolism and therefore alter the serum concentrations of hepatically metabolized AEDs. In addition, anecdotal reports suggest that several herbs and dietary supplements, such as essential oils, evening primrose and borage, and stimulants such as ephedra (ma huang) and guarana, exacerbate seizures.

Key points – non-pharmacological management

- Patients should be referred for presurgical evaluation after failure of two or more regimens using antiepileptic drugs (AEDs), particularly if they have a resectable lesion.
- Essential presurgical evaluation includes long-term video-electroencephalogram monitoring, magnetic resonance imaging with dedicated protocol, and neuropsychological assessment for language and memory functions.
- 70–80% of patients with mesial temporal sclerosis can become seizure free after anterior temporal lobectomy.
- Vagus nerve stimulation is a therapeutic option for patients with medically refractory partial-onset seizures, particularly those with non-resectable seizure foci.
- The ketogenic diet is effective adjunctive therapy for children with medically refractory epilepsy.
- The ketogenic diet should only be used under expert medical and nutritional supervision.
- Up to one-third of patients with epilepsy take herbs or dietary supplements for general maintenance of health and the control of symptoms.
- Clinicians must take a thorough history from patients regarding the use of alternative medicines, and check reliable databases for information on safety as well as possible effects on seizure frequency and AED serum concentrations.

Key references

Engel J Jr. Surgery for seizures. *N Engl J Med* 1996;334:647–52.

Engel J Jr, Wiebe S, French J et al. Practice parameter: temporal lobe and localized neocortical resections for epilepsy: report of the Quality Standards Subcommittee of the American Academy of Neurology, in association with the American Epilepsy Society and the American Association of Neurological Surgeons. *Neurology* 2003;60: 538–47; erratum 1396.

Fisher RS, Handforth A. Reassessment: vagus nerve stimulation for epilepsy: a report of the Therapeutics and Technology Assessment Subcommittee of the American Academy of Neurology. *Neurology* 1999;53:666–9.

Kossoff EH. More fat and fewer seizures: dietary therapies for epilepsy. *Lancet Neurol* 2004;3: 415–20.

National Center for Complementary and Alternative Medicine (USA). http://nccam.nih.gov/health/supplement-safety/

Peebles CT, McAuley JW, Roach J et al. Alternative medicine use by patients with epilepsy. *Epilepsy Behav* 2000;1:74–7.

Schachter SC. Vagus nerve stimulation therapy summary: five years after FDA approval. *Neurology* 2002;59(6 suppl 4):S15–20.

Schachter SC, Saper CB. Vagus nerve stimulation. *Epilepsia* 1998;39: 677–86.

Tyagi A, Delanty N. Herbal remedies, dietary supplements, and seizures. *Epilepsia* 2003;44:228–35.

Vining EP, Freeman JM, Ballaban-Gil K et al. A multicenter study of the efficacy of the ketogenic diet. *Arch Neurol* 1998;55:1433–7.

Wiebe S, Blume WT, Girvin JP et al. A randomized, controlled trial of surgery for temporal-lobe epilepsy. *N Engl J Med* 2001;345:311–18.

Wyllie E. Surgical treatment of epilepsy in children. *Pediatr Neurol* 1998;19:179–88.

Status epilepticus (SE) is a common life-threatening medical emergency characterized by frequent and/or prolonged epileptic seizures. Community-based studies in the USA suggest the incidence may be as high as 50 per 100 000 people per year, peaking in children under 1 year of age and in adults over 60 years of age. With the aging of the population, it is likely that SE will become an increasingly important public health problem.

Traditionally, SE is diagnosed when the patient has continuous or repeated seizure activity without regaining consciousness for more than 30 minutes. This time frame is defined on the basis of decompensatory cerebral damage after 30 minutes of seizure activity when physiological changes fail to compensate for the increase in cerebral metabolism. In practice, however, most authorities would recommend emergent antiepileptic drug (AED) treatment when a seizure has lasted more than 5–10 minutes, excluding simple febrile seizures.

The most readily recognized type of SE is tonic–clonic SE, but it has been estimated that approximately 25% of SE cases are 'non-convulsive' in nature. Diagnosis of the latter is established by concurrent electroencephalographic recording. Depending on the electrographic changes, non-convulsive SE is subdivided into complex partial and absence SE. SE is a neurological emergency that requires immediate treatment. SE may result from a variety of causes (Table 7.1), the commonest of which include non-compliance with antiepileptic medication, consumption of alcohol, metabolic problems, acute stroke and hypoxia.

Mortality/morbidity

Mortality and morbidity reflect the underlying cause and the physiological effects of prolonged convulsions, including hypertension, tachycardia, cardiac arrhythmias and hyperthermia. Mortality is as high as 10%, rising to 50% in elderly patients. Mortality is higher when SE is secondary to an acute insult (e.g. acute stroke, anoxia, trauma, infections, metabolic disturbance). Conversely, SE due to previous stroke, alcohol or AED withdrawal has a more favorable prognosis.

Management

Long duration of SE is associated with poor outcome. An effective management protocol should therefore be initiated immediately (Table 7.2). Any delay in treatment worsens the prognosis and reduces the likelihood of stopping seizures without having to resort to general anesthesia. The importance of a coordinated effort in the treatment of convulsive SE – involving ambulance technicians, emergency medicine specialists, medical intensivists and neurological specialists – cannot be overemphasized.

TABLE 7.1

Causes of tonic–clonic status epilepticus

With pre-existing epilepsy

Poor compliance with medication

Recent change in treatment

Barbiturate or benzodiazepine withdrawal

Presenting de novo

Presentation of a first seizure

Alcohol or drug abuse

Acute stroke

Meningoencephalitis

Acute head injury

Cerebral neoplasm

Demyelinating disorder

Metabolic disorders (e.g. renal failure, hypoglycemia, hypercalcemia)

Drug overdose (e.g. tricyclic antidepressants, phenothiazines, theophylline, isoniazid, cocaine)

Inflammatory arteritides (e.g. systemic lupus erythematosus)

Pseudostatus epilepticus

TABLE 7.2

Treatment protocol for convulsive status epilepticus (SE)

Time (min)	Action
0–5	• Diagnose SE by documentation of recurrent convulsive seizures without recovery of consciousness in between, or continuous seizure for more than 5 minutes.
	• Establish airway, and ensure adequate respiration, blood pressure and cardiac rhythm.
	• Set up i.v. line with saline. Draw blood for metabolic studies, AED levels and toxin screens.
	• Administer thiamine and glucose if indicated.
	• Give antibiotics when infection is a possibility.
5–10	• Administer either lorazepam, 0.1 mg/kg at 2 mg/min i.v., or diazepam, 0.2 mg/kg at 5 mg/min i.v.
	• Repeat once if seizure continues after 5 minutes.
	• Diazepam should be followed by i.v. fosphenytoin or phenytoin to prevent recurrence.
10–30 if SE persists	• Administer phenytoin i.v. infusion, 15–20 mg/kg, no faster than 50 mg/min in adults and 1 mg/kg/min in children.
	• ECG and blood pressure monitoring during infusion
or	• Fosphenytoin i.v. infusion, 15–20 mg PE/kg, no faster than 100 mg PE/min
or	• PB i.v. infusion, 10 mg/kg, no faster than 100 mg/min.
	• Pay special attention to respiratory depression.
30–60 if SE persists	• Administer general anesthesia with the patient intubated and under mechanical ventilation in the intensive care unit. Agents for use include pentobarbital, thiopental, propofol and midazolam.
	• Watch for potential complications associated with SE, including hypothermia, acidosis, hypotension, rhabdomyolysis, renal failure, infection and cerebral edema.
	• Continue to search for and treat any underlying cause.
	• Monitor treatment response clinically and with EEG.

AED, antiepileptic drug; ECG, electrocardiogram; EEG, electroencephalogram; i.v., intravenous; PB, phenobarbital; PE, phenytoin equivalents.

Key points – status epilepticus and seizure clusters

- Status epilepticus can be convulsive or non-convulsive.
- Emergent treatment should be given when a convulsive seizure has lasted more than 5–10 minutes.
- Poor prognostic factors include old age, acute symptomatic cause and long duration.
- Benzodiazepine administration, orally or rectally, is useful in patients experiencing clusters of seizures.

Seizure clusters

Some patients experience clusters of seizures (also called acute repetitive seizures) lasting from minutes to hours. Patients with frontal lobe epilepsy are particularly prone to clustering of seizures at night. Seizure clustering may occur around menstruation in certain women, or when patients do not take their usual AED therapy. In most cases, however, precipitating factors cannot be readily identified.

These seizure clusters may not be defined as SE but require therapeutic intervention. Acute treatment with a benzodiazepine, such as clobazam, after the first seizure can be given in an attempt to prevent further attacks. If the seizure cluster has occurred as a result of AED omission or dose reduction, reintroduction of the drug may be sufficient to abort it.

During a seizure cluster, oral therapy in a child may be problematic and intravenous access is usually unavailable or difficult. Rectal diazepam administered by parents or other caregivers may be effective in this situation. Rectal diazepam is absorbed more rapidly than rectal lorazepam or oral diazepam because of its high lipid solubility. A gel-containing, prefilled, unit-dose rectal delivery system is commercially available. The doses used in clinical studies (0.5 mg/kg for children aged 2–5 years, 0.3 mg/kg for 6–11 year olds, 0.2 mg/kg for those over 12 years of age) were effective and well tolerated, and did not produce respiratory depression. The most common side effect was somnolence. Buccal midazolam, although unlicensed, is being increasingly used in some countries instead of rectal diazepam.

Parents and caregivers must be adequately trained by knowledgeable healthcare professionals to be able to recognize seizure clusters, administer rectal diazepam, monitor the patient for potentially dangerous respiratory depression and summon emergency medical help when necessary.

Excessive usage of rectal diazepam can result in rebound seizures.

Key references

Alldredge BK, Gelb AM, Isaacs SM et al. A comparison of lorazepam, diazepam, and placebo for the treatment of out-of-hospital status epilepticus. *N Engl J Med* 2001;345: 631–7; erratum 1860.

Brodtkorb E, Aamo T, Henriksen O, Lossius R. Rectal diazepam: pitfalls of excessive use in refractory epilepsy. *Epilepsy Res* 1999;35:123–33.

DeLorenzo RJ, Hauser WA, Towne AR et al. A prospective, population-based epidemiologic study of status epilepticus in Richmond, Virginia. *Neurology* 1996;46:1029–35.

Dreifuss FE, Rosman NP, Cloyd JC et al. A comparison of rectal diazepam gel and placebo for acute repetitive seizures. *N Engl J Med* 1998;338:1869–75.

Lowenstein DH. Status epilepticus: an overview of the clinical problem. *Epilepsia* 1999;40(suppl 1):S3–8.

Mitchell WG. Status epilepticus and acute repetitive seizures in children, adolescents, and young adults: etiology, outcome, and treatment. *Epilepsia* 1996;37(suppl 1):S74–80.

Shorvon S. The management of status epilepticus. *J Neurol Neurosurg Psychiatry* 2001;70 (suppl 2):II22–7.

Treiman DM, Meyers PD, Walton NY et al. Veterans Affairs Status Epilepticus Cooperative Study Group. A comparison of four treatments for generalized status epilepticus. *N Engl J Med* 1998;339: 792–8.

Walker MC. Diagnosis and treatment of non-convulsive status epilepticus. *CNS Drugs* 2001;15:931–9.

Women of childbearing age

There are a number of specific issues relevant to women with epilepsy that are essential considerations for all doctors treating this patient population.

Contraception. Carbamazepine (CBZ), phenytoin (PHT), phenobarbital (PB), primidone (PRM), topiramate (TPM) at doses over 200 mg daily, oxcarbazepine (OXC) and felbamate (FBM) all induce the metabolism of female sex hormones. This metabolism can alter the menstrual cycle and increase turnover of the components of oral contraceptive pills and depot formulations of steroid hormones. The risk of breakthrough pregnancy is not insignificant. An oral contraceptive formulation containing 50 µg of estrogen, with subsequent adjustment depending on the presence or absence of breakthrough bleeding, can provide secure contraception. Other birth control measures must be taken until the pattern of menstruation has been stable for at least 3 months.

Levonorgestrel implants are contraindicated in women taking enzyme-inducing antiepileptic drugs (AEDs) as they have an unacceptably high failure rate. This is also likely to be the case with the progesterone-only pill. Medroxyprogesterone injections appear to be effective, though they will need to be given more frequently than is usually recommended. The morning-after contraceptive pill can be used after unprotected intercourse. The effectiveness of the hormonal method of emergency contraception is reduced by enzyme-inducing drugs; a copper intrauterine device may be offered, or the dose of levonorgestrel should be increased.

Menstruation. Up to 20% of women with epilepsy have abnormal ovarian function, including anovulatory menstrual cycles and polycystic ovaries. These problems may be more common in patients treated with sodium valproate (VPA). Some women find that their seizures worsen around menstruation, a phenomenon known as catamenial epilepsy.

This exacerbation is thought to be a consequence of imbalance between the proconvulsant estrogen and anticonvulsant progestogen concentrations. Manipulating the cycle with hormonal preparations is often unsuccessful, however, and may cause unwanted effects such as weight gain and depression. Another option is intermittent clobazam (CLB) for the few days just before and shortly after the onset of menstruation.

Pregnancy. The fertility rate of women with treated epilepsy is one-quarter to one-third lower than that of the general population. However, when women do conceive, most can expect to undergo uneventful pregnancies and deliver healthy babies. During pregnancy, metabolic processes change and close attention needs to be given to AED concentrations. Total serum concentrations of some drugs will fall, particularly those of PHT (Figure 8.1) and lamotrigine (LTG). Women whose epilepsy is well controlled usually remain seizure free during pregnancy and delivery. Conversely, those who continue to report seizures before conception may deteriorate during pregnancy.

Before conception. Although it would be ideal to withdraw AED treatment in women contemplating pregnancy, for many this would

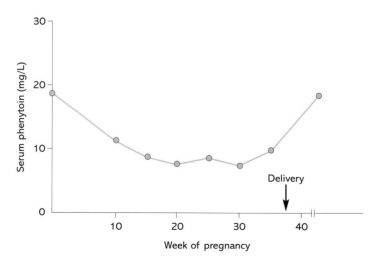

Figure 8.1 Serum phenytoin concentrations during pregnancy and delivery in a woman taking an established dose of 300 mg daily.

result in recurrence or exacerbation of seizures, which can be dangerous for both mother and baby. If the criteria for discontinuation are met (pages 51–52), the AED should be stopped over a suitable interval before conception. If AED therapy cannot be withdrawn completely, it should be tapered to a minimal effective dose of, if possible, a single drug. In addition, supplemental folic acid, 4–5 mg/day, should be administered before conception in an attempt to prevent neural tube defects. Folate treatment should be continued for the first 5 weeks of gestation, and current advice is to continue taking it at least until the end of week 12. These and other guidelines for managing epilepsy in women who are contemplating pregnancy are set out in Table 8.1.

Fetal health. The incidence of minor and major fetal malformations increases in women with epilepsy, even if they are untreated. Commonly quoted figures are 3–6% for women with epilepsy compared with 2–3% in the general population. The risk increases disproportionately with the number of AEDs taken, being approximately 3% for one drug (similar to background risk), 5% for two, 10% for three and over 20% in women taking more than three AEDs (Figure 8.2). A syndrome consisting of facial dimorphism, cleft lip and palate, cardiac defects, digital hypoplasia and nail dysplasia has been identified. This condition was initially ascribed to hydantoins including PHT (fetal hydantoin syndrome), but is now known to occur with other AEDs, including CBZ and VPA.

There are no clear data indicating differences in safety among PHT, PB and PRM. Current evidence suggests that VPA and CBZ are associated with an increased incidence of neural tube defects of about 1% and 0.5%, respectively. Preliminary results from prospective pregnancy registries suggest that the risk of major fetal malformation may be particularly high for VPA (up to 7%), but its risk may be minimized by keeping daily doses at or below 1000 mg. The teratogenic risk associated with LTG monotherapy is low, similar to that associated with CBZ. There are still insufficient data regarding the safety of other newer AEDs.

After birth. The older enzyme-inducing AEDs (CBZ, PHT, PB and PRM) can cause transient and reversible deficiency in vitamin K-dependent clotting factors in the neonate. Following a traumatic birth,

TABLE 8.1

Guidelines for managing epilepsy in women contemplating pregnancy

- After thorough discussion of the pros and cons with the woman, attempt AED withdrawal before conception if criteria are met

- If AED withdrawal is not suitable (or the woman is unwilling to attempt it), review the regimen before conception, aiming for monotherapy (if possible) with the lowest effective dose of AED; stress the importance of planned pregnancy

- Discuss the risks of seizure exacerbation as well as fetal loss, teratogenesis and development delay with the patient and her partner

- Ensure potential mothers appreciate that by the time pregnancy is confirmed, possible teratogenesis is well under way and any damage may already have been done

- Discuss available antenatal screening and the need for frequent AED measurements during pregnancy and for at least 8 weeks after delivery

- Prescribe folic acid, 4–5 mg daily, before conception and continue at least until the 12th week of gestation

- Point out the risk of hemorrhagic disorder in the newborn and the need for oral vitamin K during the last few weeks of pregnancy in women taking enzyme-inducing AEDs

- Discuss the chance of the baby developing epilepsy; children born to mothers (but not fathers) with epilepsy have a three-fold increased risk of later seizures

- Advise the patient about the need for strict AED compliance and adequate sleep throughout pregnancy

- Document each of the above in the patient's medical record

the risk of intracerebral hemorrhage increases. Accordingly, babies at risk should receive intramuscular vitamin K_1 immediately after birth, and mothers should take oral vitamin K_1, 10 mg daily, for the last few weeks of pregnancy.

After delivery, all mothers should be encouraged to breastfeed their babies. The concentrations of PHT, CBZ and VPA in breast milk are low and not usually harmful. PB, PRM and LTG can accumulate in the

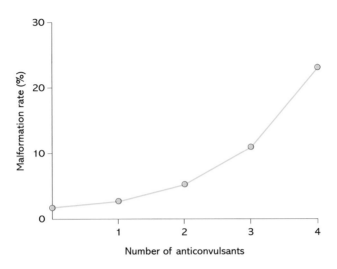

Figure 8.2 Relationship between number of antiepileptic drugs taken during the first trimester of pregnancy and the likelihood of fetal malformation. Data from Nakane et al. *Epilepsia* 1980;21:663–80.

breast-fed baby due to slow elimination. Gabapentin (GBP) and vigabatrin (VGB) are unlikely to accumulate in infants since these AEDs are excreted mainly unchanged in the urine. There are few data relating to the other newer AEDs. As a general rule, if the baby is noted to be drowsy or sedated, breastfeeding should be alternated with bottle feeding or stopped altogether.

Pregnancy registries. The Antiepileptic Drug Pregnancy Registry was established in the USA in 1996 to determine prospectively the risk of major malformations from AEDs. Women with epilepsy who become pregnant should call the toll-free number (1-888 233 2334) to enroll. Physicians cannot enroll patients; the woman herself must call as part of the informed consent process. There are three brief interviews: an initial 15 minutes, 5 minutes at 7 months' gestation and 5 minutes 2–4 weeks after birth.

In Europe, a similar project is being coordinated. This registry requires input from the attending clinician and not the patient. The European Registry of Antiepileptic Drugs and Pregnancy (EURAP) is a consortium of independent research groups that have agreed on a common protocol for a prospective assessment of pregnancy outcome. The registry has now expanded beyond Europe to include Australia, Japan and other Asian countries. All physicians who care for women taking AEDs during pregnancy are invited to contribute. They can contact their individual national coordinators or the central project commission via dbattino@istituto-besta.it.

Elderly patients

Old age is now the most common time in life to develop epilepsy. Approximately 1.5% of the population over the age of 70 years is diagnosed with active epilepsy. The number of elderly persons diagnosed with epilepsy is set to rise further with the aging of the population. Nearly all de-novo seizures in elderly people are partial in onset with or without secondary generalization. Underlying factors can be identified in a greater proportion of elderly patients than younger patients, including cerebrovascular disease, dementia and tumor. New-onset idiopathic syndromes are rare. Diagnosis of epilepsy can be challenging and may have to await a witnessed event. Complex partial seizures presenting as confusion may be misdiagnosed as psychiatric symptoms. Post-ictal confusion can be prolonged in the elderly and may contribute to physical injury sustained during a seizure.

AEDs are the mainstay of treatment, and are effective in the majority of patients. Complete seizure control can be expected in more than 70% of elderly patients. A subgroup, often with progressive neurodegenerative disease, will continue to have seizures despite all attempts at pharmacological prevention. Elderly patients are particularly sensitive to AED adverse effects, possibly because of age-related pharmacokinetic changes due to delay in gastric emptying, reduction in body fat, and decreased hepatic metabolism and renal elimination. Low doses are generally recommended in the elderly in order to minimize adverse effects.

The patient, and often the spouse and children, must be convinced of the need for lifelong treatment. Sympathetic explanation and assured support will help an elderly person regain their self-confidence after epilepsy has been diagnosed and AED treatment established. Choice of drug depends on the side-effect and interaction profiles. Drugs with a high propensity for neurotoxicity should be avoided (see Table 4.5). In patients with multiple concomitant medications, AEDs that do not produce pharmacokinetic interactions are the preferred choice (see Table 4.6). Few clinical trials of AEDs have been performed specifically in the elderly. Double-blind trials support the newer agents LTG and GBP over CBZ for the treatment of partial seizures and generalized tonic–clonic seizures, primarily because they produce fewer neurotoxic side effects. VPA is a suitable alternative as it is also well tolerated in this population and is implicated in fewer interactions than is CBZ or PHT.

Teenagers

Some types of epilepsy, such as the idiopathic syndromes juvenile myoclonic epilepsy and generalized tonic–clonic seizures upon awakening, are most likely to manifest during the teenage years. Sleep deprivation, photosensitivity and major stresses such as school examinations are common triggers. Partial seizures can also present during teenage years, either de novo or as a recurrence of a dormant childhood condition, such as mesial temporal sclerosis.

Children who develop epilepsy should be re-evaluated during their teenage years, and AED levels should be monitored. At puberty, hepatic metabolism slows to a rate approximating that of adults, which may lead to a rise in circulating AED concentrations. AED doses may, therefore, need to be reduced as a child grows older. However, such a rise is often offset by a teenage growth spurt. Falling AED levels may indicate imperfect compliance, a common occurrence in this age group.

The teenage years are an appropriate time for counseling on contraception, clarifying the possible side effects of AEDs, and predicting prognosis and eventual drug withdrawal. Driving, social interactions and career advice are other issues that doctors caring for teenagers with epilepsy must address (see Chapter 9).

Patients with learning disabilities

Epilepsy has the highest prevalence in people with learning disabilities, ranging from 5% in mildly affected individuals to 75% in those with coexisting severe cerebral palsy or postnatal brain injury. Diagnosis relies heavily on an accurate description of events, as routine investigations are rarely helpful. Tonic–clonic seizures are common, but many patients also have partial and other generalized seizure types. The clinical picture is often complicated by stereotypies and behavioral disorders. Co-prescription of antipsychotic drugs may further reduce the seizure threshold.

Before the first hospital appointment, a great deal of useful information can be obtained from a home assessment by a specialist epilepsy nurse following an agreed protocol. This assessment should include:

- description of the episodes
- evaluation of IQ
- details of concomitant medication
- previous and current AED treatment
- circulating AED levels if appropriate
- details of the carer's concerns and so on.

Home video recordings can help to confirm or refute the diagnosis of epilepsy. At the outset, a management plan, including outcome aims, should be formulated with the full involvement of the carer(s) and family. Numbers and doses of AEDs should be rationalized. Attention should be paid not only to seizure frequency and severity, but also to behavior, mood, appetite, communication, cooperation, alertness and sleep pattern. Broad-spectrum AEDs, such as VPA, LTG, TPM, zonisamide and levetiracetam, should be the preferred choice, and barbiturates and benzodiazepines should be avoided. The endpoint need not always be freedom from seizures, but perhaps better control accompanied by improved alertness, mood and cooperation.

Key points – specific populations

- Formulations containing at least 50 μg of estrogen should be used in oral contraceptives when coadministered with carbamazepine, phenytoin, phenobarbital, primidone, topiramate (TPM) (at doses over 200 mg daily), oxcarbazepine and felbamate, because these drugs induce the metabolism of female sex hormones.
- Intermittent clobazam just before and shortly after the onset of menstruation can be used in women who experience catamenial seizures.
- All established antiepileptic drugs (AEDs) are teratogenic, although the risk seems greatest with sodium valproate (VPA); the teratogenic potential of the newer drugs is unclear.
- AED treatment is continued when necessary during pregnancy on the basis that seizures, especially convulsive seizures, are more harmful to the mother and fetus than the drugs themselves; however, treatment should be tapered to a minimal effective dose before pregnancy, if possible to a single AED.
- Supplemental folic acid, 4–5 mg/day, should be administered before conception and continued at least until the end of week 12 of gestation.
- A witness's account is particularly important for the correct diagnosis of epilepsy in the elderly, in whom the presentation of seizures is often subtle.
- Low doses of AEDs are recommended in the elderly in order to minimize adverse effects, particularly neurotoxicity.
- The teenage years are an appropriate time for counseling on contraception and other lifestyle issues including driving, social interactions and careers.
- Broad-spectrum AEDs, such as VPA, lamotrigine, TPM, zonisamide and levetiracetam should be the preferred treatment choice in people with learning difficulties; barbiturates and benzodiazepines should be avoided.

Key references

Anonymous. Practice parameter: management issues for women with epilepsy (summary statement). Report of the Quality Standards Subcommittee of the American Academy of Neurology. *Neurology* 1998;51:944–8.

Arroyo S, Kramer G. Treating epilepsy in the elderly: safety considerations. *Drug Saf* 2001;24:991–1015.

Bauer J, Isojärvi JI, Herzog AG et al. Reproductive dysfunction in women with epilepsy: recommendations for evaluation and management. *J Neurol Neurosurg Psychiatry* 2002;73:121–5.

Brodie MJ, Overstall PW, Giorgi L; UK Lamotrigine Elderly Study Group. Multicentre, double-blind, randomised comparison between lamotrigine and carbamazepine in elderly patients with newly diagnosed epilepsy. *Epilepsy Res* 1999;37:81–7.

Crawford P, Appleton R, Betts T et al. The Women with Epilepsy Guidelines Development Group. Best practice guidelines for the management of women with epilepsy. *Seizure* 1999;8:201–17.

Foldvary-Schaefer N, Falcone T. Catamenial epilepsy: patho-physiology, diagnosis, and management. *Neurology* 2003; 61(6 suppl 2):S2–15.

Hannah JA, Brodie MJ. Epilepsy and learning disabilities – a challenge for the next millennium. *Seizure* 1998;7:3–13.

Rowan AJ, Ramsay RE, Collins JF et al. New onset geriatric epilepsy: a randomized study of gabapentin, lamotrigine, and carbamazepine. *Neurology* 2005;64:1868–73.

Schachter SC. Neuroendocrine aspects of epilepsy. *Neurol Clin* 1994;12:31–40.

Stephen LJ, Brodie MJ. Epilepsy in elderly people. *Lancet* 2000;355: 1441–6.

Tomson T, Perucca E, Battino D. Navigating toward fetal and maternal health: the challenge of treating epilepsy in pregnancy. *Epilepsia* 2004;45:1171–5.

Zahn CA, Morrell MJ, Collins SD et al. Management issues for women with epilepsy: a review of the literature. *Neurology* 1998;51: 949–56.

Psychiatric comorbidities

Nearly 1 in 3 patients report significant concern about their mood.
Not surprisingly then, mood states and psychiatric comorbidities
substantially contribute to the quality of life of patients with epilepsy.
The three most common psychiatric comorbidities in patients with
epilepsy are depression, anxiety and psychosis.

Depression is the most prevalent psychiatric condition in patients with
epilepsy – up to 55% of patients in some studies – and has a greater
negative impact on quality of life than seizure-specific variables such
as seizure frequency and severity.

Depression is under-recognized and, when diagnosed, often under-
treated. Depression associated with epilepsy differs clinically from
depressive disorders in non-epileptic patients. Accordingly, symptoms
of depression in patients with epilepsy often fail to meet the diagnostic
criteria for affective disorders set out in the American Psychiatric
Association's *Diagnostic and Statistical Manual of Mental Disorders
(DSM IV)*, fourth edition. Diagnosis may be further complicated
if the patient minimizes their psychiatric symptoms, or if clinicians
do not inquire about psychiatric symptoms or consider depression
to be part of the normal adaptation to the diagnosis of epilepsy.
Clinicians often inadequately treat depression because they are
concerned that antidepressant therapy will increase seizure
frequency. The consequence of under-diagnosis and under-treatment
can be fatal. The overall suicide rate in depressed patients with
epilepsy is five times higher than that in the general population
and as much as 25 times higher in patients with complex partial
seizures of temporal lobe origin.

Depression most often occurs interictally as a chronic, waxing and
waning disorder, usually in association with variable levels of irritability
and emotionality. Some patients experience depression during a
simple partial seizure (ictal depression) or during the post-ictal state.

Before initiating therapy, iatrogenic causes should be excluded. Antiepileptic drug (AED) treatment can be contributory, especially phenobarbital (PB), primidone (PRM), vigabatrin (VGB) and topiramate (TPM). Conversely, depression that follows the discontinuation of an AED with mood-stabilizing properties (e.g. lamotrigine [LTG]) can also be treated by reinstituting the AED.

Few controlled trials of antidepressants have been conducted in patients with epilepsy and depression. Selective serotonin reuptake inhibitors (SSRIs) are first-line treatments, especially citalopram and sertraline, which have minimal pharmacokinetic interactions with AEDs. Tricyclic antidepressants (TCAs) can be given as second-line therapy. Monoamine oxidase inhibitors and non-TCAs are probably best avoided. Clomipramine and lithium are more likely to worsen seizure frequency than other antidepressants. Electroconvulsive therapy is not absolutely contraindicated in patients with epilepsy but should be reserved for medication-resistant depression. In addition to antidepressants, contributing psychosocial factors should be sought and addressed by qualified professionals.

Anxiety is the second most common psychiatric condition in patients with epilepsy, with a prevalence of up to 50% in some studies. Anxiety markedly compromises quality of life and psychosocial functioning, even more so than depression in one study. Ictal anxiety may be mistaken for a panic disorder. Anxiety most commonly occurs interictally, taking the form of a generalized anxiety disorder. Severity of anxiety does not necessarily correlate with seizure frequency. SSRIs and benzodiazepines are most often used, though no controlled studies in patients with epilepsy have been reported. Some AEDs, such as sodium valproate (VPA), gabapentin and pregabalin, have anti-anxiety properties.

Psychosis. The incidence of psychosis varies according to the epilepsy syndrome, from 3.3% in patients with idiopathic generalized epilepsy to 14% in patients with temporal lobe epilepsy. Additionally, it correlates with epilepsy severity: psychosis occurs in 0.6–7% of patients with epilepsy in the community and 19–27% of epilepsy patients who require hospitalization.

Ictal psychosis presents as hallucinations or delusions. Symptoms are usually self-limiting and can be mistaken for schizophrenia or mania, but unlike a primary psychiatric disorder are associated with a pattern of non-convulsive status epilepticus on electroencephalography. Post-ictal psychosis generally begins years after the onset of epilepsy. The typical pattern is a cluster of complex partial seizures, followed by a lucid post-ictal period. In turn, this lucid period is followed by affective symptoms together with grandiose and religious delusions, as well as simple auditory hallucinations. Patients with bilateral seizure foci, bilateral limbic lesions and clusters of complex partial seizures are at particularly high risk.

Interictal psychosis manifests as delusions and hallucinations; disorganized behavior and thought disorders may also occur. Compared with patients with schizophrenia, patients with interictal psychosis have an absence of negative symptoms, better premorbid state, less deterioration of personality and better response to pharmacotherapy.

There are no controlled trials of antipsychotic or atypical antipsychotic medications in patients with epilepsy and psychosis. Haloperidol, molindone, fluphenazine, perphenazine and risperidone appear less likely to worsen seizure frequency than clozapine and loxapine. Some AEDs, such as TPM, VGB and levetiracetam (LEV), can occasionally produce psychotic reactions in susceptible patients.

Drug interactions

SSRIs, especially fluoxetine and paroxetine, may increase serum concentrations of carbamazepine (CBZ) and phenytoin (PHT). These drugs also elevate serum concentrations of TCAs.

TCAs. Serum concentrations of TCAs (which are metabolized by the 2D6 hepatic isoenzyme) are generally reduced by hepatic enzyme-inducing AEDs such as CBZ, PHT, PB and PRM. Conversely, VPA inhibits the metabolism of TCAs and, therefore, may increase their circulating concentrations.

Antipyschotics. Most antipsychotic drugs, including haloperidol, perphenazine, chlorpromazine, thioridazine, thiothixene and risperidone, are metabolized by the 2D6 and/or 3A4 hepatic isoenzymes. Serum concentrations of these drugs will, therefore, be lowered by hepatic enzyme-inducing AEDs such as CBZ, PHT, PB and PRM, and increased by VPA.

Social aspects

There are very few, if any, aspects of daily living that remain unaffected by the diagnosis of epilepsy. Restrictions on independence can be the most socially disabling – in particular the effects of epilepsy on employment, driving an automobile, life insurance and lifestyle.

Employment is important for self-esteem, supporting an independent lifestyle, and affording health insurance and the costs of epilepsy treatment. Numerous surveys show that rates of unemployment and underemployment are much higher in patients with epilepsy than in the general population. Factors most often cited are lack of available transportation (particularly if seizures preclude driving), negative attitudes of employers and employees towards epilepsy, and lack of experience in the workplace. Patients whose education was interrupted by epilepsy-related complications may need additional vocational training before they seek employment.

Clinicians should encourage their patients to work whenever possible and to recommend they seek legal help if they encounter discrimination in the workplace. In the USA, the Americans with Disabilities Act protects a person from being denied employment because of a medical condition if that person can perform the essential duties of that job. In the UK, in line with several other European countries, a similar Disabilities Discrimination Act was introduced in 1995 to protect people with disabilities from discrimination in employment. Whether patients should disclose their epilepsy before being hired is best dealt with on a case-by-case basis.

Driving an automobile is often viewed as essential to holding a job and living independently. However, since driving is a privilege, applicants must meet the requirements established by their state, province or country to qualify for a driver's license. With reference to epilepsy, these requirements usually specify a seizure-free interval necessary for driving, the obligations of the patient and the physician to notify the authorities of the patient's status, and allowances that are made under certain circumstances, such as seizures that only occur during sleep or seizures that occur during a physician-prescribed AED taper. Clinicians should be thoroughly familiar with the applicable laws where they practice, and should clearly document their discussions with patients. Clinicians should also remember that side effects of AEDs, especially sedation, may interfere with a patient's ability to safely operate an automobile, and should advise patients accordingly.

Life insurance. Patients with epilepsy may be unable to find affordable life insurance, particularly if applying for an individual policy. Most insurance companies ascribe a globally higher risk of mortality to people with seizures, irrespective of the applicant's frequency or severity of seizures. Patients who obtain life insurance through their place of employment generally do not have a problem.

Lifestyle considerations. Clinicians should counsel patients on lifestyle modifications that reduce the risk of provoking seizures and help maintain overall health without unduly limiting activities that bring enjoyment and fulfillment. Reducing or eliminating the consumption of alcohol, engaging in stress-reducing behaviors, eating regularly and getting adequate sleep help reduce seizure frequency. Regular aerobic exercise, especially conducted in such a way that having a seizure would not pose a safety risk, is important for general maintenance of health as well as bone health. Participation in organized sports is generally possible, though the possibility of concussions should be minimized and athletes should consider discussing their condition with team trainers and doctors in advance.

Key points – quality of life

- Depression and anxiety are common in patients with epilepsy, and have a significantly negative impact on quality of life.
- The potential benefit of treating depression and anxiety pharmacologically outweighs the risk of increased seizures.
- Psychosis is uncommon in patients with epilepsy, and generally occurs following a cluster of complex partial seizures.
- When psychotropic medications and antiepileptic drugs are coadministered, dosages may need to be adjusted because of potential pharmacokinetic interactions.
- Patients should be encouraged to work whenever possible, and to seek legal help if they encounter discrimination in the workplace.
- Legal restrictions on driving for people with epilepsy vary; clinicians should be aware of the relevant laws in their place of practice, and must clearly document their discussion with patients.
- Patients with epilepsy may have difficulties in finding affordable life insurance.
- Patients should be counseled on lifestyle modifications that reduce the risk of provoking seizures without unduly limiting activities.

Key references

Cramer JA, Blum D, Reed M, Fanning K; Epilepsy Impact Project Group. The influence of comorbid depression on quality of life for people with epilepsy. *Epilepsy Behav* 2003;4:515–21.

Fisher RS, Vickrey BG, Gibson P et al. The impact of epilepsy from the patient's perspective I. Descriptions and subjective perceptions. *Epilepsy Res* 2000;41:39–51.

Gilliam F, Kuzniecky R, Faught E et al. Patient-validated content of epilepsy-specific quality-of-life measurement. *Epilepsia* 1997;38: 233–6.

Goldstein MA, Harden CL. Epilepsy and anxiety. *Epilepsy Behav* 2000;1: 228–34.

Hausman SV, Luckstein RR, Zwygart AM et al. Epilepsy education: a nursing perspective. *Mayo Clin Proc* 1996;71:1114–17.

Kanner AM. Psychosis of epilepsy: a neurologist's perspective. *Epilepsy Behav* 2000;1:219–27.

Koch-Stoecker S. Antipsychotic drugs and epilepsy: indications and treatment guidelines. *Epilepsia* 2002;43(suppl 2):19–24.

Lehrner J, Kalchmayr R, Serles W et al. Health-related quality of life (HRQOL), activity of daily living (ADL) and depressive mood disorder in temporal lobe epilepsy patients. *Seizure* 1999;8:88–92.

Nakken KO. Physical exercise in outpatients with epilepsy. *Epilepsia* 1999;40:643–51.

Perrine K, Hermann BP, Meador KJ et al. The relationship of neuropsychological functioning to quality of life in epilepsy. *Arch Neurol* 1995;52:997–1003.

Schmitz B. Antidepressant drugs: indications and guidelines for use in epilepsy. *Epilepsia* 2002;43(suppl 2): 14–18.

Torta R, Keller R. Behavioral, psychotic, and anxiety disorders in epilepsy: etiology, clinical features, and therapeutic implications. *Epilepsia* 1999;40(suppl 10):S2–20.

A change in approach

With the recent introduction of a broad range of new antiepileptic drugs (AEDs) that convey differing, sometimes single and often multiple, mechanisms of action, there is an imperative to replace the largely empirical approach to the pharmacological management of epilepsy with a more science-based rationale governing drug choice. Linked to this must be a better understanding of how seizures are generated and propagated in the brains of individual patients to provide classifications that have a neurobiological rather than an observational basis. These developments will underpin a patient-centered, mechanistic approach to the management of epilepsy. Combining drugs with complementary modes of action has the potential to improve the unsatisfactory prognosis for some people with refractory epilepsy. However, we also need to develop drugs with novel pharmacological properties, in particular, to revitalize the management of the malignant encephalopathic syndromes of early childhood, such as Lennox–Gastaut syndrome and infantile spasms. Current therapy aims to prevent seizures; future treatments should influence the natural history of the epileptic process.

Genetic progress

The prospect of predicting drug response based on individual genotype offers the possibility of significant health benefits to patients. The genetics underlying a range of epilepsies are beginning to yield their secrets. This approach will contribute substantially to the refinement of the seizure and syndrome classifications, and encourage AED development based on pharmacogenomics. The introduction of 'gene therapy' for the progressive myoclonic epilepsies and other devastating syndromes is a long-term goal that requires a better understanding of their functional bases. Pharmacogenomics may also offer other therapeutic opportunities, such as reversal of drug transporter activity within the blood–brain barrier and around lesional epilepsies, which have been implicated in the development of pharmacoresistance. The long-term hope is that the most appropriate AED for an individual patient could be identified with a single, straightforward DNA test undertaken at the time of diagnosis.

Surgical intervention

Surgery is considered the treatment of choice for many patients with lesional epilepsies. This must be performed early before the deleterious effects of repeated seizures produce irreversible neuronal damage, cognitive impairment and psychosocial dysfunction. Epilepsy surgery has been shown to be cost-effective compared with lifelong treatment with one or more of the newer AEDs. Advances in brain imaging are increasingly able to identify patients suitable for surgery early in the course of the disorder and also help to delineate more precisely the target area for resection. A range of brain stimulation techniques are being devised for patients resistant to AED therapy and not suitable for surgery. It may soon be possible, for instance, to increase inhibition or damp down excitation in an epileptic focus by local release of small amounts of a drug in response to burst firing in a coterie of dysfunctioning neurons.

Continued advances

Advances in the understanding, investigation and treatment of epilepsy are continuing apace. Many more people with epilepsy can expect to have their seizures controlled pharmacologically without debilitating side effects. A wider range of medical and surgical strategies are becoming available to optimize treatment for patients with more severe seizure disorders. The development of potentially revolutionary therapies will require close liaison between scientists and clinicians to coordinate theory with implementation, thereby improving the lives of many more people with epilepsy over the next decade.

Useful resources

Management guidelines

American Academy of Neurology

www.aan.com/professionals/
practice/guideline

1. Evaluating a first non-febrile seizure in children
2. Treatment of the child with a first unprovoked seizure
3. Reassessment: vagus nerve stimulation for epilepsy
4. Management issues for women with epilepsy
5. Neuroimaging in the emergency patient presenting with seizure
6. Efficacy and tolerability of the new antiepileptic drugs I: Treatment of new onset epilepsy
7. Efficacy and tolerability of the new antiepileptic drugs II: Treatment of refractory epilepsy
8. Temporal lobe and localized neocortical resections for epilepsy
9. The use of felbamate in the treatment of patients with intractable epilepsy

Other guidelines

Crawford P, Appleton R, Betts T et al. The Women with Epilepsy Guidelines Development Group. Best practice guidelines for the management of women with epilepsy. *Seizure* 1999;8:201–17.

Epilepsy Foundation of America's Working Group on Status Epilepticus. Treatment of convulsive status epilepticus. *JAMA* 1993;270: 854–9.

Karceski S, Morrell MJ, Carpenter D. Treatment of epilepsy in adults: expert opinion, 2005. *Epilepsy Behav* 2005;7(suppl 1):S1–S64.

Koch-Stoecker S. Antipsychotic drugs and epilepsy: indications and treatment guidelines. *Epilepsia* 2002;43(suppl 2):19–24.

National Institute for Clinical Excellence. Newer drugs for epilepsy in adults. London: NICE, 2004. www.nice.org.uk/TA076guidance

Scottish Intercollegiate Guidelines Network. Clinical guideline (CG) 70: Diagnosis and management of epilepsy in adults. 2003; CG 81: Diagnosis and management of epilepsies in children and young people. 2005. www.sign.ac.uk.

Schmitz B. Antidepressant drugs: indications and guidelines for use in epilepsy. *Epilepsia* 2002;43 (suppl 2):14–8.

Professional organizations

American Academy of Neurology
1080 Montreal Avenue
Saint Paul, MN 55116
Tel: 800 879 1960 or
+1 651 695 2717
Fax: +1 651 695 2791
memberservices@aan.com
www.aan.com
Practice guidelines are available at:
www.aan.com/professionals/
practice/guideline

American Epilepsy Society
342 North Main Street
West Hartford, CT 06117-2507
Tel: +1 860 586 7505
Fax: +1 860 586 7550
www.aesnet.org

Association of British Neurologists
Ormond House
27 Boswell Street
London WC1N 3JZ
Tel: +44 (0)20 7405 4060
Fax: +44 (0)20 7405 4070
info@theabn.org
www.theabn.org

British Paediatric Neurology Association
204 Greenmount Lane
Heaton, Bolton BL1 5HZ
Tel: +44 (0)1204 491171
info@bpna.org.uk
www.bpna.org.uk

European Epilepsy Academy
EUREPA Secretariat
Maraweg 21
D-33617 Bielefeld
Germany
Tel: +49 (0)521 144 4310
Fax: +49 (0)521 144 4311
office@epilepsy-academy.org
www.epilepsy-academy.org

International League Against Epilepsy
Avenue Marcel Thiry 204
B-1200 Brussels, Belgium
Tel: + 32 (0)2 774 9547
Fax: + 32 (0)2 774 9690
www.ilae-epilepsy.org

Patient Support Groups

Asian and Oceanian Epilepsy Association
www.aoea-online.org

Epilepsy Action (UK)
(British Epilepsy Association)
New Anstey House
Gate Way Drive
Yeadon
Leeds LS19 7XY
Tel: +44 (0)113 210 8800
Fax: +44 (0)113 391 0300
Helpline: 0808 800 5050
helpline@epilepsy.org.uk
epilepsy@epilepsy.org.uk
www.epilepsy.org.uk

Epilepsy Foundation (USA)
4351 Garden City Drive
Landover, MD 20785-7223
Tel: +1 800 332 1000
www.epilepsyfoundation.org

The Epilepsy Therapy Development
Project (USA)
11921 Freedom Drive, Suite 730
Reston, VA 20190
Tel: +1 703 437 4250
Fax: +1 703 437 4288
epilepsycure@aol.com
www.epilepsy.com
www.epilepsy.com/professionals
www.epilepsyproject.org

International Bureau for Epilepsy
Stichting Epilepsie Instellingen
Nederland
PO Box 21, 2100 AA Heemstede
The Netherlands
Tel: +31 (0)23 55 88 412
Fax: +31 (0)23 55 88 419
hdboer@seinl.nl
www.ibe-epilepsy.org

Joint Epilepsy Council of the UK
and Ireland
(Umbrella body for epilepsy
organizations)
PO Box 186
Leeds LS20 8WY
Tel: +44 (0)1943 871852
www.jointepilepsycouncil.org.uk

National Centre for Young People
with Epilepsy (UK)
(Major provider of specialized care
to young people with epilepsy in
the UK)
St Piers Lane
Lingfield
Surrey RH7 6PW
Tel: +44 (0)1342 832243
info@ncype.org.uk
www.ncype.org.uk

National Society for Epilepsy (UK)
Chesham Lane
Chalfont St Peter
Bucks SL9 0RJ
Tel: +44 (0)1494 601300
Helpline: +44 (0)1494 601400
www.epilepsynse.org.uk

SUDEP, Epilepsy Bereaved (UK)
(The UK's leading organization on
sudden unexpected death in
epilepsy and epilepsy-related death)
PO Box 112
Wantage
Oxon OX12 8XT
Tel: +44 (0)1235 772850
Bereavement line: +44 (0)1235
772852
epilepsybereaved@dial.pipex.com
www.sudep.org

Index

FAST FACTS

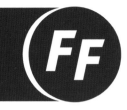

An outstandingly successful independent medical handbook series

Over one million copies sold

- Written by world experts
- Concise and practical
- Up to date
- Designed for ease of reading and reference
- Copiously illustrated with useful photographs, diagrams and charts

Our aim for *Fast Facts* is to be **the world's most respected medical handbook series**. Feedback on how to make titles even more useful is always welcome (feedback@fastfacts.com).

Fast Facts titles include

Acne
Allergic Rhinitis
Asthma
Benign Gynecological Disease (second edition)
Benign Prostatic Hyperplasia (fifth edition)
Bipolar Disorder
Bladder Cancer
Bleeding Disorders
Brain Tumors
Breast Cancer (third edition)
Celiac Disease
Chronic Obstructive Pulmonary Disease
Colorectal Cancer (second edition)
Contraception (second edition)
Dementia
Depression (second edition)
Disorders of the Hair and Scalp
Dyspepsia (second edition)
Eczema and Contact Dermatitis
Endometriosis (second edition)
Erectile Dysfunction (third edition)
Gynecological Oncology
Headaches (second edition)

Hyperlipidemia (third edition)
Hypertension (second edition)
Inflammatory Bowel Disease
Irritable Bowel Syndrome (second edition)
Menopause (second edition)
Minor Surgery
Multiple Sclerosis
Osteoporosis (fourth edition)
Parkinson's Disease
Prostate cancer (fourth edition)
Psoriasis (second edition)
Respiratory Tract Infection (second edition)
Rheumatoid Arthritis
Schizophrenia (second edition)
Sexual Dysfunction
Sexually Transmitted Infections
Skin Cancer
Smoking Cessation
Soft Tissue Rheumatology
Superficial Fungal Infections
Travel Medicine
Urinary Continence (second edition)
Urinary Stones

Orders

To order via the website, or to find regional distributors, please go to
www.fastfacts.com

For telephone orders, please call +44 (0)1752 202301 (Europe),
800 247 6553 (USA, toll free) or 419 281 1802 (Canada)